Acupressure: simple steps to health

15

By the same author:

Vital Energy: Oriental Exercises for Health and Well-Being
Self-Massage
Cystitis: Comprehensive Guide to Effective Treatment
Eastern Healing: The Practical Guide to the Healing Traditions
of China, India, Tibet & Japan
Rainbow Bridge: A Spiritual Odyssey

Acupressure:
simple steps to health

Discover Your Body's Powerpoints for Health and Relaxation

Jacqueline Young

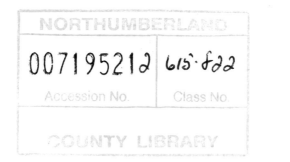

Thorsons

Thorsons
An Imprint of HarperCollins*Publishers*
77–85 Fulham Palace Road,
Hammersmith, London W6 8JB

The Thorsons website address is:
www.thorsons.com

and *Thorsons*

are trademarks of
HarperCollins *Publishers* Limited

Originally published as *Acupressure for Health* by Thorsons 1994
Then as *Acupressure Step by Step* by Thorsons 1998
This edition published by Thorsons 2001

10 9 8 7 6 5 4 3 2 1

© Jacqueline Young 1994

Jacqueline Young asserts the moral right to
be identified as the author of this work

A catalogue record for this book
is available from the British Library

ISBN 0 00 712002 8

Photography by Dave King
Text illustrations by PCA

Printed and bound in Great Britain by
Scotprint, Haddington, East Lothian

Dedication

For my mother and stepfather, Joosje and Don Angel – for all their loving support.

For all the participants at my acupressure classes and clinics;
I have so much enjoyed sharing and learning together.

And for all those who read this book: may you gain many
benefits from the practice of acupressure.

About the Author

Jacqueline Young is an acupuncturist, clinical psychologist and writer who lived for many years in the Far East studying and practising Oriental medicine and health-care techniques. She is a visiting lecturer at several colleges of acupuncture and massage in the UK and Europe and a popular presenter of public workshops on acupressure, Oriental exercises and other self-help therapies. The author of several books and many articles on natural medicine, she also has a clinical practice in central London.

For information on her classes and publications, please send a s.a.e. to Health Systems, PO Box 2211, Barnet, Herts, EN5 4QW, UK, or access www.jacquelineyoung.com

Contents

Part 2: Acupressure Health Workout

Chapter 1: Acupressure Health Workout 15–37

Part 3: Acupressure Health

Chapter 2: The Head 41–108

Chapter 3: The Joints 109–34

Part 4: Acupressure First Aid

Appendices:

Acknowledgements

With thanks to all those who have masterminded this completely new edition of *Acupressure: Simple Steps to Health* and to all those who have written to me after reading earlier editions. I am so delighted to know that the acupressure techniques described in this book are helping you to better health. Keep those letters coming!

To all those new to acupressure may this book help and inspire you on your path to health and happiness.

This new edition is offered with thanks to all my teachers, clients and students and is dedicated to the memory of the late Cecil Saker – an extraordinary man.

Jacqueline Young, London 2001.

This book is different from previous acupressure books written for the lay public in that it focuses on health and preventive health care rather than just on disease. It clearly describes how to balance acupressure points, what the correct sensation is, and how much pressure to apply. It also explains the principles of direction of flow of *chi* along the meridians and includes complementary techniques such as breathing and visualization, both of which quite definitely affect the flow of chi.

It is an eminently practical book and is very simply set out, with very clear photos and diagrams on what points to use to both optimise health and to treat a whole range of conditions. It can be used perfectly easily without reading the whole book by simply reading the introduction, then looking up your area of concern in the index and turning up the particular part of the book which tells you how to approach it from an acupressure point of view. In each section there is an explanation as to what the points are actually doing, so making this discipline more understandable to the Western mind. This is of great importance, as the concepts underlying acupuncture and acupressure are foreign to the Western mind, making it difficult for us to think in terms of energy and flow of energy around the body. We are culturally pre-programmed to think in terms of organs that we can actually see.

Jacqueline Young has produced an eminently readable text which will be of benefit to anyone who buys this book.

Julian Kenyon, M.D., M.B., Ch.B.
Medical Director, The Dove Clinic for Integrated Medicine, London.

part one

Introduction

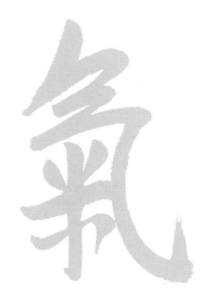

Introduction

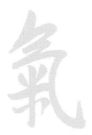

Nowadays there is so much you can do to help yourself to health and to stay healthy. Both ancient and modern wisdom and techniques for promoting health are widely available to guide us along the path. Modern research has demonstrated the importance of diet and nutrition, for example the importance of balancing proteins, carbohydrates and other foods and of reducing fats, or the effects of specific vitamins and minerals. Similarly, sports science has clearly demonstrated the importance of regular exercise, and it is now possible to know exactly how to combine different types of exercise and training for peak fitness. Work in psychophysiology and psychology has clearly shown the effects of stress on both the physical body and on the mental state: performance is impaired, chemical changes occur, concentration deteriorates and a sense of well-being is lost. This work has led to the development of a range of psychological techniques to promote both mental and physical health–techniques for relaxation, stress management, positive thinking and attitudinal change.

As we assimilate this wide range of knowledge and experience and try to put it into practice in our daily lives, our attention must also be drawn to the wonderful range of self-care practices advocated by ancient healing traditions. These traditions were based not on scientific research, but rather on long and patient observation of the natural cycles in nature and the rhythms of life. All the ancient Oriental medical systems of China, Japan, India, Tibet and Korea advocate thorough self-care regimes as preventive medicine and as a curative approach for simple health problems. In the same way, the Western traditions of folk and herbal medicine have always recommended specific actions alongside the ingestion or application of remedies in order to prevent ill-health and bring about cure.

Within the Oriental systems a common theme is the importance of the flow of 'vital energy' (known as *chi* or *qi* in Chinese and *ki* in Japanese) in the body to promote and prolong health. When this flow is blocked or depleted there is ill-health; when it flows freely and abundantly there is good health and well-being. The supply and flow of this vital energy, which courses through invisible channels in the body known as 'meridians', is dependent on diet, life-style, environment, posture, breathing, habits, body movement and exercise, mental attitude, personality and spirit. As a result, self-care approaches emphasize the importance of eating foods according to the seasons and according to what suits your physical constitution and body type. They also recommend behavioural changes such as the need to live a balanced life-style with regular sleep and exercise, living in a moderate environment (avoiding extremes of temperature for example), and the importance of keeping good company. There are also a wide range of exercises for promoting the flow of energy within the body and for both calming and strengthening the mind and spirit, leading to increased mental powers and heightened awareness.

One of the simplest and most effective of these techniques is acupressure, the application of fingertip or thumb pressure at specific points on the body (known as 'acupoints') to stimulate meridian flow and internal organ function in order to promote health and prevent, or ease, health imbalances. The technique dates back thousands of years and is both safe and effective. Acupressure is easy to learn and takes only a short time to apply. It is also very cost-effective as it requires no special equipment, creams or other materials, just a pair of hands and a developing sense of touch in order to locate the point accurately and determine the effect of acupressure on it.

Acupoints are located all over the body, close to the surface of the skin, and are linked together in a complex network of meridian channels. Each acupoint has specific effects on individual organs or body systems. Stimulating, or gently massaging, the points triggers a response within the meridians that leads to direct physiological changes in the body and can affect mental and emotional states too.

acupressure
simple steps
to health

This book describes the acupressure technique, how it works and how it can be used to promote health as well as to prevent or relieve a wide range of common ailments. It gives clear descriptions of the location of each acupressure point, the techniques for applying acupressure and the functions of the points. It shows how to promote health

in all the major body systems and organs and also links this with simple self-health techniques, including breathing, diet, nutrition, exercise, life-style, mental attitude and visualization, in order to provide an integrated approach to health in body, mind and spirit. The book is designed to appeal to all those interested in promoting and maintaining their own health and helping others do the same.

Acupressure for Health

Acupressure's real use is as a health-care, self-care technique for *promoting* health balance and *preventing* disease and disorders. It can also be used as an effective tool for easing and curing common, minor ailments or as an adjunct to therapy for more serious conditions.

In line with this tradition, the focus of this book is therefore on health rather than on disease. It starts with a complete Acupressure Workout for promoting vitality and good health in the whole body. This routine can be performed daily and used to maintain good health and prevent disease. There are then sections focusing on each part and system of the body, showing how acupressure can be used to optimize body functions and well-being. Contained within each of these sections are general health-care tips[1] and also acupressure prescriptions for preventing and relieving common disorders.

Acupressure, used wisely, can give you real power at your fingertips: the power to promote your own health, to detect imbalances at an early stage through self-awareness and the ability to restore balance. However, acupressure is not a substitute for medical treatment in the case of serious illness, so if your symptoms persist or you are unsure what is causing them, you should always seek medical advice.

If you are in poor health, or have a chronic health problem, acupressure can be used in conjunction with whatever treatment you are currently receiving to assist the body in gradually restoring its natural healing mechanisms and good health.

---

1. Throughout the text there is reference to various vitamins and minerals. Ideally, consult a nutrition book (see Further Reading) or a nutritionist (see Useful Addresses) for information on the best food sources of each. Alternatively, they may be taken as supplements but, again, get advice from a specialist on dosage, consumption, etc.

DISCOVERING ACUPOINTS AND THEIR EFFECTIVENESS

Many years ago, before I had even heard of acupuncture or trained as an acupuncturist myself, I suffered from very bad low back pain. I used to rub my lower back to ease the pain and eventually began to notice that some particular spots were more tender than others. Pressing on these points felt comfortable and seemed to bring some relief. Gradually, I also noticed that at certain times, for example during menstruation or colds, other particular parts or points on the body also became more sensitive than usual.

To my great surprise, over a decade later when I began to study acupuncture, I found that many of these sensitive points corresponded exactly to the locations of specific acupoints. As I had already experienced their effectiveness for myself, I began to experiment further with acupressure. I also shared the technique with others and was able to witness their surprise and satisfaction at their health improvement. Later I started to use acupressure in my clinical practice and found that not only was it excellent as a therapy in its own right, especially for those who were apprehensive about acupuncture needles or very sensitive, weak or frail, but it was also very effective when practised by patients themselves in between treatments. It enabled them to play an active part in their treatment and also often led to a reduction in the number of treatments required. Many continued to use acupressure to maintain and further improve their health after treatment had finished.

In my many years of clinical work I have given large numbers of clients acupressure points to use between treatments and to promote their general health and vitality. Their encouraging feedback and the good results they obtained, with very little effort or training, led me to establish classes and workshops in acupressure for both lay people and health professionals. These classes have now been offered in many different countries, and also with groups of children, the disabled and the elderly. Seeing the enjoyment and positive effect that participants gained from this powerful form of self-care led to the writing of this book.

The Acupoints

An acupoint is a point of increased sensitivity and powerful effect located along an acupuncture meridian. There are over 360 acupoints located on the meridians all over the body and new acupoints are constantly being discovered. Individual acupoints have a direct and specific effect on individual organs or body systems and some are more powerful, or potent, than others; it is these major points that are most commonly used during acupressure. This acupressure book includes around 100 of the acupoints that are considered most effective for promoting health and preventing or relieving common ailments. It also describes many combinations of points that are known to aid health balance. Some acupoints are local to the body part or organ which they regulate, while others are located on a different part of the body and affect the specific body part or organ from a distance.

The acupoints are numbered and named according to the meridian on which they are located and its corresponding internal organ. Most are bilateral, occurring on *both sides* of the body, so acupressure must be applied to both points of the pair. Other points, located on the midline of the body or spine, are single points.

LOCATING THE ACUPOINTS

The exact location of each acupoint is described in terms of the part of the body, where it is located and its position relative to the bones, muscles or tendons. Most acupoints are located in small depressions, or hollows, on the body in between bones, muscles or tendons. Each location description is accompanied by a drawing or photograph.

After following the descriptions closely and paying careful attention to the illustrations, spend a little time feeling around the area with your most sensitive finger to locate the point accurately. There is almost always a slight sensitivity or 'charge' to be felt at the site of an acupoint and, in the case of imbalance, the point itself is often tender. The points are generally located with the tip of the index or middle finger or the thumb. With regular practice, sensitivity develops and confidence increases. As you become more practised it will become easier and easier to locate acupoints correctly on both yourself and others.

Technique

Each acupoint has a correct technique for locating the point and for applying pressure. Usually the same fingertip or thumb used to locate the point is used to apply pressure. Sometimes the nail edge is used and it should be clean and smooth. Pressure is applied gently at first and gradually increased to the point where mild sensation, but not pain, is felt. In healthy people, or those with strong constitutions, quite firm, direct pressure may be required before sensation is felt. For sensitive individuals, infants, the elderly or those who are weak or frail, only very light stimulation is required.

Acupressure is either applied in a sustained way or intermittently by locating the point, applying pressure, releasing, relaxing and repeating the sequence several times. Additional stimulation can also be given by applying gentle, small massage rotations to the point. Never force the pressure or strain the muscles, as this will lead to aching and tension in the hands, wrists and shoulders. Always ensure that your body is in a comfortable position and relaxed, then locate the point with the fingertip, nail edge or thumb and slowly and gently apply pressure accompanied with relaxed breathing. Release the point gently when you have finished, breathe out and relax the body.

Some people experience acupressure as a dull aching or a slight 'electrical' sensation, that often peaks and then disappears. If you experience this, then the moment at which the sensation disappears is the time to stop applying acupressure, as this indicates that a balancing has already occurred. You should also stop or ease the pressure if at any time the acupressure becomes painful. Otherwise, continue applying the acupressure for 30 seconds to 2 minutes, or whatever feels comfortable for you.

ACUPRESSURE BALANCING

Acupressure can be used in different ways to balance the body. If there is little sensation and a feeling of 'emptiness' at an acupoint then slow, gentle pressure should be used at first and gradually built up over a minute or two while you breathe deeply, emphasizing the in-breath. If the sensation at an acupoint is strong and tender, then more vigorous, light but firm acupressure should be applied for a shorter period of time (around 30 seconds to 1 minute) and the focus is more on breathing out than in.

Remember to locate and apply pressure to the acupoint on both sides of the body except for points on the Conception and Governor Vessel meridians, on the mid-line of the body and the spine, and on certain of the 'extra' points. Note the difference in sensation as you massage each side and alternate the side on which you start.

ACUPOINT SENSATION

The amount of sensation at an acupoint may vary. A strong sensation is usually a sign of excess or over-function while little, or no, sensation signifies deficiency and weakness.

Excess conditions usually involve pain, swelling, inflammation or acute symptoms. Deficient conditions are characterized by fatigue, weakness, aching and long-standing illness. The causes of excess or deficient conditions may be poor diet, faulty posture, stress, mental anxiety or faulty life-style habits, including overwork and lack of exercise and sleep. Acupressure can help to restore balance by regulating the flow of vital energy in the body and improving internal organ function.

If the sensation is different on either side of the body for a pair of bilateral points, then first apply acupressure to the side that feels more comfortable and less tender. As balance is restored, the sensation at the 2 bilateral acupoints will gradually become more similar.

Sensitivity at acupoints also varies slightly according to other factors such as the menstrual cycle or weather conditions. Being alert and noting how these sensations change will teach you a lot about your state of health.

AMOUNT OF PRESSURE

Use light pressure when you feel weak or tired and, as already mentioned, on those who are frail, sensitive, elderly or infants. Also use light pressure when pregnant or on those suffering from high blood pressure. Otherwise, firm pressure can be used and should be applied by leaning in with body weight rather than forcing with the muscles. Fleshy parts of the body can take more pressure than bony parts or the face.

DIRECTION OF FLOW

The direction for the application of acupressure is very important. Generally, you are advised to work in the direction of flow of the acupuncture meridian on which the point is located, as this helps to improve the vital energy flow within the meridian and enhance the function of the corresponding internal organ. Occasionally, pressure is applied perpendicularly or even in the opposite direction to the flow in order to have a sedative and calming effect. However, if in doubt, go with the flow, as traditional theory maintains that this enhances the natural homoeostatic function of the body and promotes health in whatever way the body requires. This process is further helped by correct breathing and visualization.

BREATHING

It is important to be in a relaxed and comfortable position during acupressure and to maintain relaxed, full, breathing throughout. Generally, acupressure is applied during exhalation as this helps to tonify and activate the acupoint. In cases of severe pain, swelling or inflammation, however, you may get better results if the acupressure is applied on inhalation as this helps to sedate the point and can lead to a reduction in symptoms.

VISUALIZATION

Acupressure can be even more effective when it is accompanied by clear, positive visualization. If you know the location of the meridian channels, then visualize vital energy flowing along them as you stimulate the acupoint. Also visualize the organ you are connecting with as healthy and functioning well and, if you are using acupressure to relieve a particular ailment, visualize the condition as improving and cured. For example, if you are using acupoints to enhance respiratory function, visualize the lungs as strong and healthy and all respiratory functions working well while you apply the acupressure. If using the acupoints to relieve, say, a cold or cough, then clearly visualize normal function being restored to the lungs and nasal passages and the condition having cleared. Deep, full breathing accompanying the visualization enhances both clarity and concentration and seems to increase effectiveness.

SELECTING ACUPOINTS

Combinations of acupoints are given here that promote health in each body part and system. Additional acupoints are suggested for the prevention and relief of particular ailments. You do not always have to use all the points. Use your own sensitivity and awareness to determine which points are the most effective for you and concentrate on them. Some people get better results with more points and some with fewer, so you are your own best guide. Apply acupressure to the acupoints in the order given, which corresponds to the order of acupoints in a given meridian, the traditional order of flow between meridians, or sequencing according to the part of the body where the point is located and its effects. Generally, acupressure is applied from the top of the body to the bottom and from the front to the back, as this has a relaxing and balancing effect.

Practice

WHO CAN PRACTISE?

Acupressure is safe, effective and suitable for anyone; all you need is the willingness to learn and practice. It can be effectively used by both lay people and health professionals as an adjunct to therapy and can be applied at any age or stage of life from babies to the elderly. However, remember always to start with light pressure in order to gauge sensitivity and body reactions to the acupoint. Also remember to take careful note of the cautions and contraindications in the text.

WHEN TO PRACTISE

Acupressure can be practised anytime, anywhere, but it is advisable not to do it directly after eating or when very hungry or tired. Allow at least an hour after eating a meal or take a light snack or rest first. It is best if you are comfortable and relaxed and, if possible, in a quiet, warm and well-ventilated room. In good weather acupressure can also be practised out of doors.

HOW LONG TO PRACTISE

The length of the time that acupressure is applied will depend on individual sensitivity and the degree of health or imbalance. Generally, application for 1–3 minutes is sufficient, and little and often is more effective than a longer period at irregular intervals. In the case of an acute condition, or profound discomfort or pain, acupressure should be repeated regularly throughout the day at hourly or 2-hourly intervals, then gradually decreased to 3 times a day as the condition improves and finally 2–3 times a week to maintain improvement and prevent recurrence. For long-standing conditions, regular acupressure 2–3 times a week over several weeks or months should lead to improvement. The Acupressure Health Workout (see pp. 15–37) and the Facial Workout (see pp. 41–58) are effective when used 2–3 times a week.

PREPARATION

Before you begin acupressure, take a few minutes to stretch and relax the body, breathe deeply and release any mental tension or worry. Loosen any tight clothing, get in a comfortable position and rub the hands together to warm them. Rotate the wrists and flex the hands and individual fingers to increase circulation in them.

Performing Acupressure on Others

As you become increasingly confident and competent you will be able to start locating acupoints on others. You can help them improve their health, relieve common ailments and learn to use this self-health technique for themselves. You can also ask others to give acupressure to you. This is relaxing and enjoyable and helpful for acupoints that are difficult to reach, such as those on the back.

WORKING WITH CHILDREN, THE ELDERLY AND THE DISABLED

Children have a natural talent for acupressure. They find it easy to locate the acupoints, enjoy receiving acupressure, are good at positive visualization and have no difficulty in accepting its effectiveness. Acupressure is also a powerful self-help tool for those with disabilities and can be an enjoyable and helpful form of interaction when applied by someone else. The elderly can also benefit considerably as acupressure can help to mobilize joints, relieve pains or discomfort and maintain good health and well-being.

Contraindications

Acupressure should not be used when a person is under the influence of alcohol or non-medicinal drugs. Great care should also be taken if the person is extremely weak, sensitive or fatigued, in which case only light pressure should be used until strength and vitality have been built up.

Strong pressure should also be avoided on all points during pregnancy especially Large Intestine 4, Spleen 6 and Urinary Bladder 60 (see notes in the text) as these points are used to facilitate labour and birth. For these points just lightly touch with the fingertips or thumb and focus on breathing and visualization.

Acupressure should never be applied directly on cuts, wounds, scars, bruises or veins. Instead it should be applied *around* these sites of injury.

Consulting a Specialist

The acupressure techniques described in this book can be safely used by anyone to maintain and promote health as well as to relieve common ailments or for use in first-aid situations. However, acupressure does not replace conventional diagnosis and treatment in the case of serious health problems. If any health condition persists, or worries you unduly, you should consult a medical or complementary practitioner for professional advice. In addition, if you are using acupressure during pregnancy, labour or post-partum care it would be advisable to do so in conjunction with an experienced acupuncturist or acupressure practitioner who could help you monitor your progress.

Research

There is an increasing body of research underway which supports acupressure's effectiveness. This research shows that stimulation of acupoints can lead to a wide range of physiological changes including: electrical changes in the skin at acupoint sites; changes in brain chemicals, such as increased release of endorphins (the body's natural pain killers); and altered internal organ function such as changes in heart or respiration rates (see Further Reading). It is clear that this simple technique can indeed have a profound, wide-ranging effect on the body.

How to Use this Book

Begin by reading this introduction thoroughly as it contains important information on the technique and application of acupressure. Then start by familiarizing yourself with the Acupressure Workout (pp. 15–37), which can immediately be put to daily use to promote your general health. Once you are comfortable with the Acupressure Workout, you can add the Facial Workout if you wish (pp. 41–58) and select acupoint combinations from the rest of the text according to the body part or system you wish to improve or the ailment you wish to prevent or relieve.

Each part of the body is covered in order from the head to the toes. Ailments are listed alphabetically in the index at the back of the book. Keep a regular diary to note your progress with acupressure.

Motivation and Confidence

Start practising acupressure today! Don't let doubt or lack of confidence distract you. As your desire to maintain regular practice and your confidence increase, so will the effectiveness of the technique. It is your participation, as much as the technique itself, that makes acupressure a success.

Your efforts with acupressure can lead to substantial changes in your life, including increased vitality and confidence and improved health. By adding positive thoughts, the mind becomes comfortable and peaceful. Slowing and deepening the breath increases oxygenation of the tissues and a sense of well-being prevails. As well-being increases, so does the feeling of harmony with others and the desire to help others. According to traditional Chinese medical theory, as the mind is rested internally and the senses focused deeply, so too the vital energy of the body and one's spirit are nourished. Acupressure can play a part in this process.

part two

Acupressure
Health **Workout**

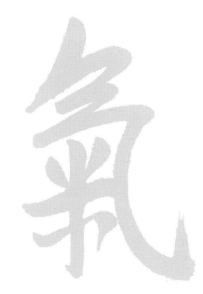

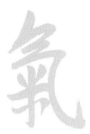

To give your body an overall tone-up, and to promote general good health and vitality, this complete Acupressure Workout can be done morning and evening or whenever you have spare time.

The routine consists of acupressure to one or more of the major acupoints on each meridian in the order of the flow of energy along the meridians. By stimulating these points, every part of the body, internal organ and major body system is energized.

This routine can be easily learnt and safely practised by anyone, although there are certain points which should not be given strong acupressure during pregnancy. (These are generally points which are used to assist labour.) Such points are clearly marked with a caution in the text. Instead of using acupressure, pregnant women can just lightly touch the relevant points with the fingertips and, taking a couple of gentle, deep breaths at each point, visualize vital energy gently suffusing the meridians.

As for all acupressure, your fingertip or thumb pressure should be firm and even. You should feel the sensation of pressure or tingling but not pain. Remember to apply pressure perpendicularly below the skin, or angled slightly in the direction of flow of the meridian, to breathe deeply and evenly and to visualize energy flowing into the meridian and appropriate body parts.

Each time you practise this workout, focus awareness on the different sensations at your fingertips and in your body. Notice how sensations change each day and also any changes in your physical health. It is quite normal for sensations to vary according to the weather, diet, environment and menstrual cycle. For example, women tend to feel more skin sensitivity around the time of their periods, certain foods may increase skin sensitivity and skin sensations may be heightened during stormy weather because of the electrical charges built up in the atmosphere. By increasing your awareness of the body's responses to different situations such as these you will develop a fine understanding of how your body works and how to take care of it.

This workout can be performed standing or sitting on the floor, on a bed or in a chair. Follow the order given below. Take your time and stay relaxed, breathing freely throughout. The complete workout should take 15–20 minutes, but you can make it last longer if you wish by spending more time focusing on your breathing and visualization at every point.

To Start

- First stretch your body and take a couple of deep breaths.

- Make sure you are relaxed and comfortable and free your mind of any mental worries.

- Don't perform the workout directly after eating or when very hungry or exhausted. Take a light snack or some rest first.

- Rub the palms together and do a few gentle finger and hand stretches and wrist exercises to loosen up before starting.

- Loosen any tight clothing, get in a comfortable position and rub the hands together to warm them.

Work through the points in the order shown below. Remember to apply pressure to points on both sides of the body except for the Conception and Governor Vessel points on the front and back midline of the body. Begin by applying the acupressure to each point on the *left* side of the body first and then on the right. The next time you practise, apply the acupressure to each point on the *right* side of the body first and then on the left.

Alternating the side that you start with in this way will help to maintain balance in the body. Check regularly during your practice that you are still relaxed, comfortable and breathing deeply.

Remember to always locate the point correctly first and then apply pressure.

The Workout

1. Lung 7: The Respiratory System

Location: On the inside of the wrist, 2 finger widths from the wrist crease closest to the palm on the same side as the thumb in the depression behind the bone.

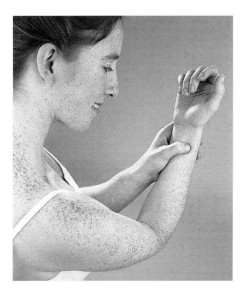

Technique: Using the thumb of the opposite hand, touch the point and then gently begin to apply pressure below the skin, angled slightly down towards the wrist and thumb. Apply sustained pressure or small, massage rotations to the acupoint. Use the fingers of the same hand under the wrist as support. Continue to apply pressure for 30 seconds to 1 minute while breathing rhythmically and visualizing the lungs as healthy and strong. Repeat on the opposite wrist.

Benefits: Strengthens the respiratory system. Helps to prevent and alleviate colds, coughs, congestion and breathing difficulties.

2. Large Intestine 4: The Head, Face and Skin

Location: In the centre of the triangle made between the small bones of the index finger and thumb. Can also be located at the end of the crease made by the index finger and thumb when they are pressed together.

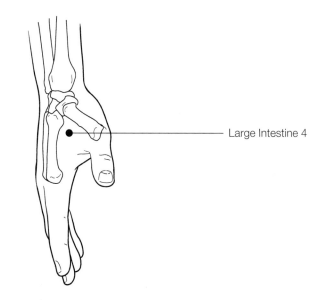

Large Intestine 4

Technique: Locate the point and then press in gently with the thumb of the opposite hand, placing the fingers underneath the acupoint, against the palm of the hand, for support. Press deeply and perpendicularly into the point, applying sustained pressure or small massage rotations to the acupoint for 30 seconds to 1 minute. Breathe deeply and visualize the whole of the upper body being filled with vitality. Repeat on the opposite hand.

Benefits: This point benefits the whole upper body. In particular it helps tone the skin and improve the complexion. It aids large intestine function, facilitating elimination and thereby helping to improve the skin quality and texture. It can be useful in relieving con-stipation and can also improve mobility and relieve pain in the arms, shoulders and neck.

Note: If pregnant, see pp. 10–11.

3. Large Intestine 11: The Arms, Skin and Digestion

Location: When the elbow is bent the point is located in the depression at the end of the skin crease towards the outside of the elbow.

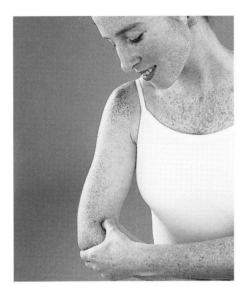

Technique: Support the elbow in the fingers and palm of the opposite hand. Press in deeply with the thumb for 30 seconds to 1 minute, applying sustained pressure or small massage rotations to the acupoint with relaxed, even breathing. Visualize healthy, clear skin and good function of the large intestine. Repeat on the opposite elbow.

Benefits: Used in conjunction with *Large Intestine 4*, this point also tones the skin, improves the complexion, ensures strong, healthy function of the large intestine and aids elbow and arm mobility. In addition, it is effective in preventing or relieving constipation.

| # 4. Stomach 36: The Digestive System

Location: Four finger widths below the lower edge of the kneecap in the hollow between the 2 bones of the leg.

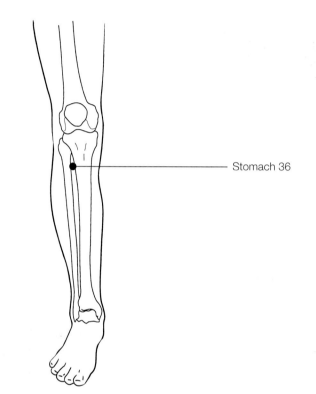

Stomach 36

Technique: Using the thumb, locate the point and apply sustained pressure or small massage rotations to the acupoint, angled slightly downwards towards the feet. Place the fingers behind the knee for support.

Alternatively, reverse the position of the hand and press with the index or middle fingers. Apply pressure for 30 seconds to 1 minute and visualize the digestive organs as healthy and strong. A tingling sensation may be felt down into the toes. Repeat on the other leg or, if you wish, acupressure can be applied to both legs simultaneously.

Benefits: Strengthens and improves digestion. Can prevent and relieve constipation, diarrhoea and indigestion. Helps build stamina.

5. Spleen 6: The Digestive System and Gynaecological Organs

Location: Four finger widths above the tip of the ankle bone in the middle of the inside of the leg.

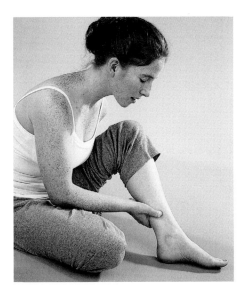

Technique: Measure 4 finger widths up from the ankle bone with one hand and then use the thumb of the other hand to locate the acupoint. Apply pressure perpendicularly or use small massage rotations to the acupoint for 30 seconds to 1 minute. Repeat on other leg.

Benefits: This very powerful acupoint is the meeting point of the Spleen, Liver and Kidney meridians. Acupressure to this point helps digestion and can relieve abdominal bloating and loose stools. It tones and strengthens the gynaecological organs and helps to keep them in position, i.e. regular acupressure is said to prevent uterine prolapse and hernia.

For women this acupoint is useful in regulating menstruation, and acupressure in the week prior to each menses can help prevent period pains and premenstrual tension. However, this point is contraindicated during pregnancy as it can induce labour (see pp. 10–11). For men this point is said to increase virility and can prevent seminal emission and relieve pain in the genital organs.

Acupressure of this point can also be used to improve mobility and relieve pain in the lower extremities.

6. Heart 7: Circulation and Heart Function

Location: With your palm upwards, this point is located on the outside edge of the first crease closest to the palm of the wrist, in the hollow level with the little finger.

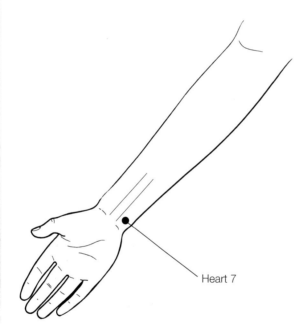

Heart 7

Technique: Support the wrist with the fingers of the opposite hand and locate the point with the thumb. Apply pressure with the thumb in the direction of the little finger for 30 seconds to 1 minute. Use sustained pressure or small, massage rotations. Repeat on the opposite wrist.

Benefits: Improves circulation, strengthens heart function and calms the mind and is very effective in relieving anxiety and insomnia. Can be used to ease mild chest pain and palpitations, though if these symptoms persist, you should always consult a medical practitioner.

7. Small Intestine 3: The Head, Neck and Spine

Location: Make a loose fist. The point is located in the middle of the longest crease on the outside edge of the little finger, just below the knuckle.

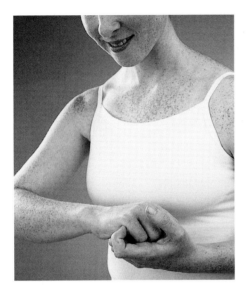

Technique: Support the fist with the fingers of the opposite hand and press into the point lightly with the edge of the nail of the thumb or forefinger. For general toning, press for 30 seconds to 1 minute but, should you be suffering from acute neck, shoulder or spinal pain, continue for 2–3 minutes and repeat every half-hour until the pain starts to ease off. Repeat on the opposite hand.

Benefits: This acupoint has a powerful connection with the back. It helps to strengthen the spine and neck and also clears the head. It can be used to prevent and ease headaches and to relieve tension or pain in the neck, shoulders and back.

8. Urinary Bladder 11: Bones

Location: At the back of the neck in line with the shoulders and level with the lower edge of the first thoracic vertebra. Located 2 finger widths on either side of the spine.

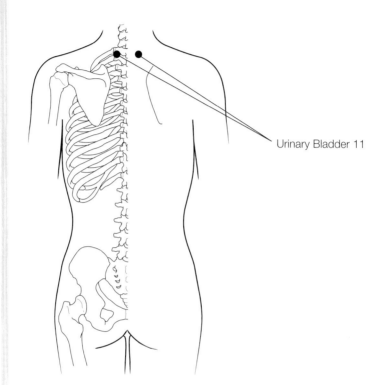

Urinary Bladder 11

Technique: Reach the hands over the back on either side of the neck and apply firm, relaxed pressure to the points with the index or middle fingers for 30 seconds to 1 minute. Both points can be stimulated simultaneously, using sustained pressure or small massage rotations. Breathe evenly and visualize healthy, strong bones throughout the body. If your arms become tired, lower them for a moment and then repeat. You should experience mild tingling under your fingertips and an enjoyable sensation of the relief of any tension in this area.

Benefits: Regular acupressure to this point on both sides of the spine is said to promote strong, healthy bones throughout the body. It can also help prevent and relieve neck and shoulder pain and tension headaches.

Location: In between the tendons at the back of the knee when the knee is slightly bent.

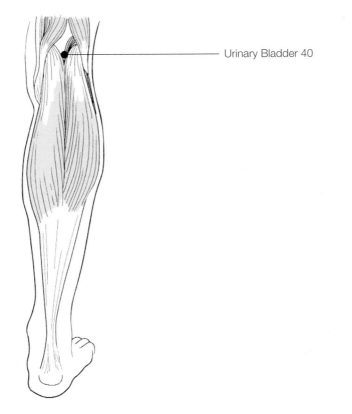

Urinary Bladder 40

Technique: Place the thumbs on the outside of each kneecap and the fingers behind the knees, while bending the knees slightly. Use the middle or index fingers of each hand to locate the hollow between the tendons at the back of each knee. Don't press on the tendons themselves and avoid varicose veins, if you have any. Apply firm, even pressure for 30 seconds to 1 minute, breathing deeply and visualizing energy flowing freely throughout the lower body. Both points can be massaged simultaneously.

If you are applying acupressure to this point on someone else, sit in front of them, place your fingers round the back of their knees with the thumbs at the sides for support, locate the point and apply pressure with the middle or index fingers. While doing so, ask the person to practise the breathing and visualization.

Benefits: Helps to promote circulation and the flow of vital energy throughout the lower body. Can improve mobility of the back and legs and relieve aching, pain or stiffness in these areas.

10. Urinary Bladder 60: Back, Legs and Feet and Urinary System

Location: In the hollow behind the ankle bone on the outer side of the foot.

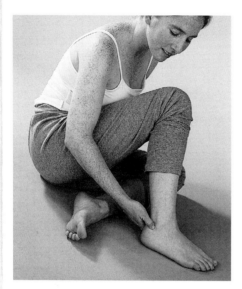

Technique: Locate the point with the thumb, using the index finger for support on the other side of the ankle. Alternatively, the position of the thumb and index finger can be reversed and the index finger used to apply acupressure to the point. Apply acupressure for 30 seconds to 1 minute, using sustained pressure or small firm rotations angled slightly downwards towards the heel. Repeat on the opposite ankle. Breathe deeply and visualize a good flow of energy through the back, legs and feet and a healthy urinary system.

Benefits: Strengthens the urinary system and improves mobility in the back, legs and feet. Can help prevent and relieve mild urinary infections, headaches, eye problems, back pain, ankle stiffness and pain in the feet.

Note: If pregnant, see pp. 10–11.

11. Kidney 1: Vitality and Blood Pressure

Location: A third of the way down the sole of the foot, in the depression just below the ball of the foot.

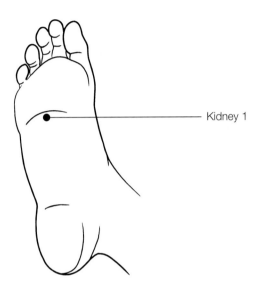

Kidney 1

Technique: Turn the foot over or outwards, resting it in the fingers of the hand on the same side of the body. Use the thumbs to locate and apply pressure to the acupoint on the soles of alternate feet or both feet simultaneously for 30 seconds to 1 minute. Use sustained pressure or apply small massage rotations to the acupoint. In cases of blood pressure problems, apply only light pressure. Breathe deeply and visualize vital energy flowing throughout the body and healthy kidneys.

Benefits: Promotes vitality and stimulates the flow of energy throughout the body. Relieves fatigue and acts as a natural stimulant. Helps to balance blood pressure, prevents and relieves dizziness and faintness and stimulates kidney function.

12. Kidney 3: Urinary System, Adrenals and Gynaecological Organs

Location: On the inside of the ankle in the hollow halfway between the ankle bone and the back of the ankle, level with the ankle bone.

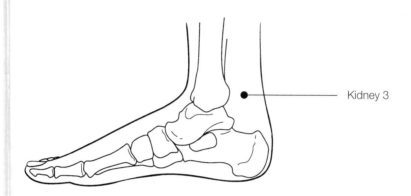

Kidney 3

Technique: Place the fingers of the opposite hand behind the ankle for support and locate the point with the thumb. Apply pressure perpendicularly for about 30 seconds to 1 minute, using sustained pressure or small rotations angled slightly upwards towards the shin. Alternatively, place the middle or index fingers on *Urinary Bladder 60* and the thumbs on *Kidney 3* and massage both points on both ankles simultaneously. Breathe freely and visualize healthy and vital urinary and gynaecological organs.

Benefits: Strengthens the kidneys, adrenals, urinary bladder and gynaecological organs and promotes good hormonal balance. Can prevent or relieve insomnia, asthma, sore throats, ear problems, toothache and low back pain.

For women, can help regulate menses and prevent menstrual problems. For men, can strengthen sexual function and treat impotence and premature ejaculation.

Location: Between the tendons on the inside of the arm, 3 finger widths above the wrist crease closest to the palm.

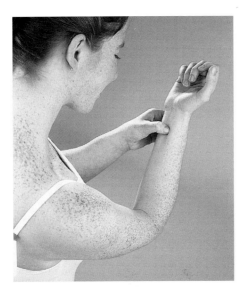

Technique: After measuring up the arm, rest the wrist in the fingers of the other hand and use the thumb to locate the point. Apply gentle pressure angled slightly downwards towards the palm and middle finger for 30 seconds to 1 minute. Breathe evenly and deeply and visualize good heart function and circulation of blood and energy throughout the upper body. Repeat on the opposite arm.

Benefits: Stimulates and regulates heart function and promotes good circulation of blood and energy throughout the arms and upper body. Can prevent or relieve mild chest or gastric pain, nausea and travel sickness, and pain or stiffness in the wrist and elbow.

14. Triple Heater 5: Circulation and Balance

Location: On the outside of the forearm, 3 finger widths above the wrist in the hollow between the bones.

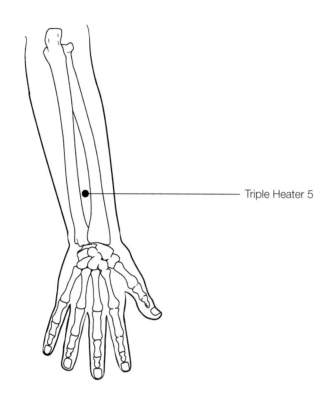

Triple Heater 5

Technique: After measuring up the outside of the arm, rest the wrist in the fingers of the other hand and use the thumb to locate and apply pressure to the acupoint for 30 seconds to 1 minute. Breathe deeply and visualize good circulation throughout the body and an even balance between the 3 areas of the body: upper, middle and lower. Repeat on the opposite arm.

Benefits: Promotes circulation through the whole body and a good balance in function and vitality between the upper, middle and lower body and the vital organs contained in each of these areas. Can prevent or relieve fevers, headaches, ear problems and pain in the elbow, wrist or fingers.

15. Gall Bladder 34: Muscular System

Location: On the outside of the leg in the hollow just beneath the meeting point of the 2 leg bones, 1 thumb width above and 2 finger widths to the outside of *Stomach 36*.

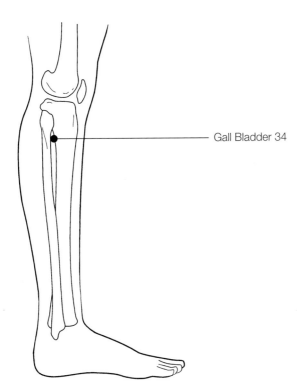

Gall Bladder 34

Technique: Place the fingers round the outsides of the legs, just below the knees, and locate the point on both legs, using the thumbs. Apply firm pressure with the thumbs angled downwards towards the feet. Maintain pressure for 30 seconds to 1 minute, using sustained pressure or gentle rotations of the thumbs. Breathe freely and visualize strong, flexible muscles throughout the body.

Benefits: Nourishes the muscles and tendons by improving the flow of blood. Promotes general mobility in the lower body and can relieve numbness and pain in the legs and feet. Also promotes good functioning of the gall bladder and liver and can relieve pain in the area of the lower ribs.

16. Liver 3: Nervous and Immune Systems

Location: On the top of the foot in the web between the first and second toes, just before the join of the small bones of the foot.

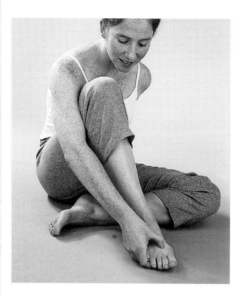

Technique: Place the fingers under the foot for support and apply acupressure to the point perpendicularly with the thumb. Take care to press in the hollow between the bones and tendons rather than on the tendons or blood vessels themselves. Use sustained pressure or small rotations. Apply pressure for 30 seconds to 1 minute, breathing evenly and visualizing a healthy liver, balanced nervous system and strong immune system. Repeat on the other foot.

Benefits: This point calms the nervous system and strengthens the liver and immune system. It can also help prevent or relieve headaches, dizziness, cramps in the foot or lower leg and breast pains.

Location: Just below the nose, in the middle of the groove above the upper lip.

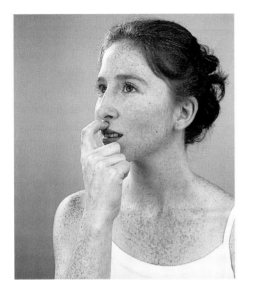

Technique: Take the fingertip or nail of the index or middle finger and apply gentle pressure perpendicularly for about 30 seconds. Breathe freely and visualize a clear mind with sharp mental function.

Caution: Take care not to stimulate this point too hard if you have high blood pressure; stop immediately if you feel unwell or uncomfortable.

Benefits: Stimulates mental alertness and brain function and aids concentration and memory. Can prevent or relieve faintness and ease back pain.

18. Conception Vessel 6: Abdominal Tonic

Location: Two finger widths below the navel on the midline of the abdomen.

Technique: Use 2 fingers to measure down from the navel and locate the point. Apply pressure gently with the middle or index finger of the other hand for about 30 seconds. Use gentle, rotating movements and apply the pressure directly into the abdomen, below the surface of the skin. Allow your breathing to become slow and relaxed and visualize warmth and power filling the abdomen.

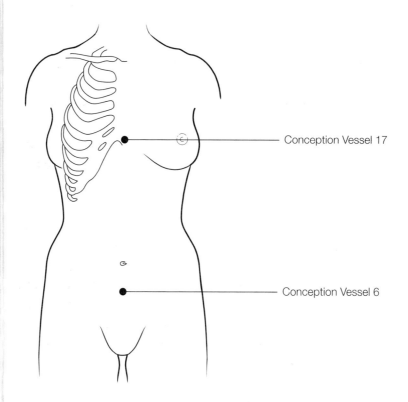

Conception Vessel 17

Conception Vessel 6

Benefits: This is one of the most important toning points for the whole body but, in particular, it strengthens the sexual organs and helps builds stamina, confidence and vitality. Regular acupressure applied to this point can prevent or relieve fatigue, menstrual problems and urinary weakness.

19. Conception Vessel 17: Upper Body Tonic

Location: In the middle of the chest in line with the nipples.

Technique: Locate the point with the middle or index finger and apply pressure gently for 30 seconds to 1 minute. Breathe deeply and evenly and visualize a good flow of energy and a powerful supply of oxygen from the lungs suffusing the chest and upper body.

Benefits: This powerful point promotes healthy function of the heart and lungs and vitality in the upper body. It can also prevent or relieve chest pain, asthma and hiccoughs.

20. Ear Massage: Lymph and Hormonal Systems

To complete this workout, spend 30 seconds to 1 minute applying acupressure to each ear. The ear is filled with hundreds of tiny micro-acupoints that correspond to every part of the body. Ear acupressure therefore applies a general stimulus to all the internal organs and body systems helping to bring them into balance. It also helps to stimulate the lymph and hormonal systems and boost immunity.

Use the nail of either the index or middle fingers, ensuring that the nail edges are smooth and clean. First apply gentle pressure on the outside edges of the ears, working from the base of the earlobes up to the tops of the ears and placing the thumbs behind the ears for support. (The thumbs should move with the fingernails so that they are always at the back of the ear supporting the pressure applied with the nails). Use light, gentle movements that feel comfortable. Breathe normally and visualize good health and vitality throughout the whole body. Then repeat the movement on the inner surface of the ears, again working from the base up to the top.

Ear acupressure is an ideal way to complete your Acupressure Workout. It can also be used on its own at any time of the day to refresh and invigorate.

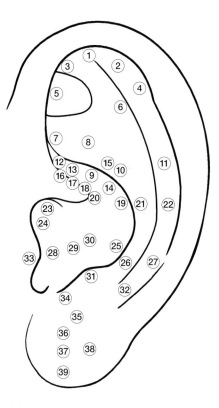

Acupoints of the ear showing corresponding internal organs.

1. Toe
2. Finger
3. Ankle
4. Wrist
5. Uterus
6. Knee
7. Pelvis
8. Buttock
9. Gall Bladder
10. Abdomen
11. Elbow
12. Urinary Bladder
13. Kidney
14. Pancreas
15. Lower Back
16. Large Intestine
17. Appendix
18. Small Intestine
19. Liver
20. Stomach
21. Chest
22. Shoulder
23. Oesophagus
24. Mouth
25. Spleen
26. Neck
27. Shoulder Joint
28. Trachea
29. Heart
30. Lung (round both sides of heart)
31. Brain Point
32. Clavicle
33. Nose
34. Testis (ovary)
35. Forehead
36. Tongue
37. Eye
38. Internal Ear
39. Tonsil

To Finish

At the end of the workout, stretch the arms above the head, stretch the back and legs and take a deep breath in. Breathe out as you relax the stretch. Repeat 3 times.

Shake out the hands and wrists to make sure they are relaxed. If you have been applying relaxed pressure your fingers should not feel tired or ache. In the beginning, however, when you are not used to the technique, it is easy to apply too much pressure or to have tension in the hands and fingers, causing them to ache afterwards. If you do have this problem, gently stretch each finger and, next time you do the workout, use lighter pressure and constantly check to make sure there is no tension in the hands.

At the end of the workout you should feel refreshed and vitalized in mind and body and all your internal organs will have been primed to function well. With practice you will be able to remember the points easily and will no longer need to keep referring to the text. This will enable your movements to be more flowing and your breathing rhythmical.

Regular use of this Acupressure Workout should lead you to feel both more energetic and relaxed. You will probably notice a decrease in minor ailments and an enhanced sense of well-being. Give the workout a try on a daily basis for a month and judge the results for yourself.

As you become more proficient your self-awareness and sensitivity will increase, making the workout even more effective. This will also enable you to select acupoints from other sections in this book, as appropriate, with skill and confidence.

part three

Acupressure
Health

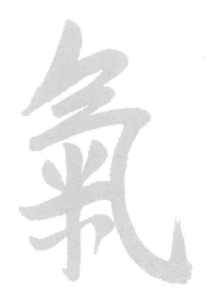

In this section each part and major system of the body is covered in turn, along with mental and emotional states. For each, the acupoints that optimize health are given, together with general natural health-care tips as appropriate. Common disorders are also included, with acupoints for both preventing and relieving them.

Once you are familiar with the Acupressure Workout described in Chapter 1, you can start to select acupoints from the following sections according to the part or system of the body that you wish to strengthen, or the disorder that you wish to alleviate.

The points are best used to maximize health and to *prevent* disease, but they can also be used in conjunction with treatment or medication, whether complementary or orthodox, to speed recovery. However, if you have an acute infection or serious health problem or are pregnant, do seek the advice of a practitioner experienced in acupressure (see Useful Addresses section) to guide you in your selection and use of points. Acupressure is not dangerous and does not have side-effects, but the points do have powerful effects on the body and should be used wisely.

Do keep a brief acupressure diary to record your practice and progress so that you can accurately assess the effects of your acupressure and develop your skill. Record how you feel, the acupoints you use and the effects you observe after and between each treatment.

Acupressure is a joy to use and, as you become convinced of its effectiveness, it will become an essential part of your own health care.

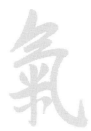

The Face and Skin

Acupressure can be used as a simple, natural and effective facial health routine to enhance the complexion, firm and tone facial skin and muscles, enhance the function of the eyes, ears and nose and improve the health of the teeth and gums.

Facial Workout

For a complete 'facial workout', apply acupressure to the following set of 20 facial points in the order shown. (These acupoints can also be combined together with simple massage techniques to form a comprehensive and effective facial massage routine, as outlined in my book *Self-Massage*.)

Regular use of this facial sequence, together with sensible diet, exercise and sleep, and lots of water will make your face and skin positively glow with health!

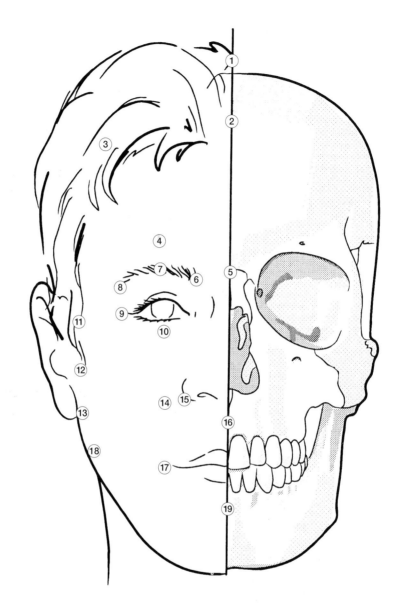

1. Governor Vessel 20
2. Governor Vessel 23
3. Stomach 8
4. Gall Bladder 14
5. Forehead (Extra)
6. Urinary Bladder 2
7. Eyebrow (Extra)
8. Triple Heater 23
9. Gall Bladder 1
10. Stomach 1

11. Triple Heater 21
12. Small Intestine 19
13. Gall Bladder 2
14. Stomach 3
15. Large Intestine 20
16. Governor Vessel 26
17. Stomach 4
18. Stomach 6
19. Conception Vessel 24
20. Gall Bladder 20 (see pp. 57–58)

Technique: The acupressure techniques for the face are just the same as for the Acupressure Workout. Use your index finger, middle finger or thumb to apply acupressure to each of the points, either perpendicularly below the surface of the skin or else with gentle, circular pressure angled slightly in the direction of flow of the meridian.

Acupressure can be applied to most of the facial acupoints on both sides of the face simultaneously. Pressure should be firm but light, especially around the eyes, and should be maintained for short periods at first. Begin with around 5 seconds for each point and build up to 10 seconds if you wish. Overall, the feeling should be comfortable and refreshing. Let your facial feeling guide your technique.

The facial acupressure points, in order of use, are as follows:

1. Governor Vessel 20

Location: At the top of the head on the midline between the tops of the 2 ears and in line with the top of the nose. Locate the point by placing the thumbs on the top of each ear and stretching the middle fingers out to meet at the top of the head.

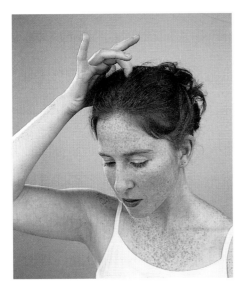

acupressure

the head

Technique: Apply acupressure perpendicularly into the scalp, using the middle or index fingertip of one hand. For firmer pressure you can rest the middle or index fingertip of the other hand on top of the nail of the finger locating the point and apply gentle pressure with both fingers simultaneously. The point should be felt as a small depression in the scalp and may feel slightly tender. **Do not overstimulate this point if you have high blood pressure.**

Benefits: Improves mental clarity, brightens the face and complexion, enhances the eyes and drainage in the nasal passages.

2. Governor Vessel 23

Location: About 1 finger width inside the hairline on the midline of the scalp in line with the top of the nose.

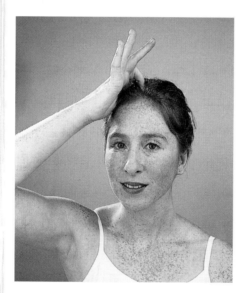

Technique: Apply acupressure perpendicularly, using the middle or index fingertip as for the previous acupoint. Rest the thumb on the temple at the side of the head for support.

Benefits: Clears the head and enhances the eyes.

3. Stomach 8

Location: At the corner of the forehead, 1 finger width inside the hairline.

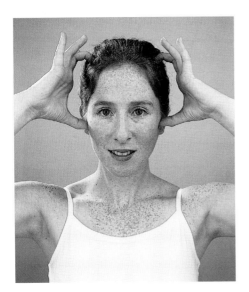

Technique: Rest the thumbs at the sides of the cheeks for support and locate the acupoint on both sides of the forehead using the middle or index fingers. Apply acupressure perpendicularly, pressing into the scalp.

Benefits: Relieves tension in the head and improves eye function.

4. Gall Bladder 14

Location: On the forehead about 1 thumb width above the middle of the eyebrows.

Technique: Place the thumbs against the temples for support and locate the points on both sides of the forehead simultaneously, using the middle or index fingers. Apply acupressure perpendicularly or angling slightly upwards towards the hairline.

Benefits: Smooths and clears the forehead, relieving any tension. Relieves tension or pain in the eyes.

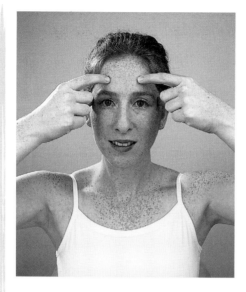

5. Forehead Point (Extra Point)

Location: Above the bridge of the nose halfway between the inner edge of each eyebrow.

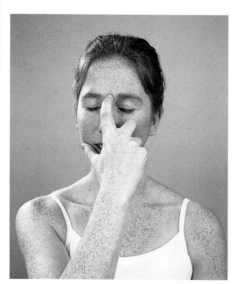

Technique: Locate with the index or middle fingertip, resting the thumb against the side of the face for support. Apply acupressure perpendicularly or angled slightly downwards towards the bridge of the nose.

Benefits: Releases tension in the forehead and clears the nasal passages.

6. Urinary Bladder 2

Location: On the inner edge of the eyebrow, above the inner corner of each eye.

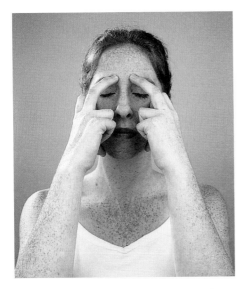

Technique: Locate the acupoint with the thumbs, resting the fingers lightly on the forehead for support or, alternatively, use the middle or index fingertips with the thumbs against the jaw for support. Angle the pressure upwards against the bony socket above the eyes.

Benefits: Brightens the eyes and clears the nasal passages.

7. Eyebrow Point (Extra Point)

Location: In the middle of the eyebrow, directly above the pupil of the eye.

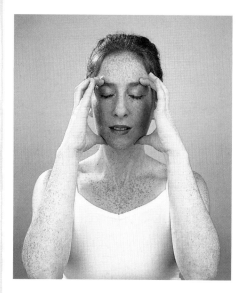

Technique: Resting the thumbs under the chin for support, locate the acupoint using the middle or index fingers. Apply acupressure against the bony sockets. Apply pressure to both points simultaneously.

Benefits: Relieves eye tension and pain.

8. Triple Heater 23

Location: In the depression at the outer edge of the eyebrow.

Technique: Place the thumbs under the jaw-bone for support and locate the acupoint with the index or middle fingers. Apply acupressure against the bony sockets and angled in slightly towards the eyebrow. Stimulate both points simultaneously.

Benefits: Increases circulation around the eye and improves eye function. Tones the skin around the eyes.

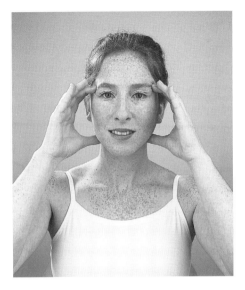

9. Gall Bladder 1

Location: In the depression level with the outside corner of the eye.

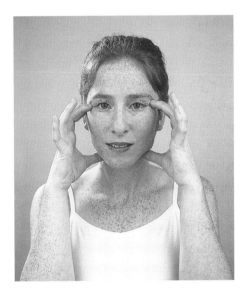

Technique: Resting the thumbs against the jaw-bone for support, locate the acupoint with the index or middle fingers and apply acupressure angled slightly away from the eye. If you wish, you can also move the fingertips 1 finger width outwards towards the ears, and raise them slightly so that they are halfway between the outer edge of the eye and the eyebrow and apply acupressure at this site. This is another Extra Point, the *Temple* acupoint (see p. 68). Apply pressure to both sides simultaneously.

Benefits: Improves eyesight and relieves tension in forehead.

10. Stomach 1

Location: Directly below the pupil of the eye, in the middle of the ridge of the bony socket below the eye.

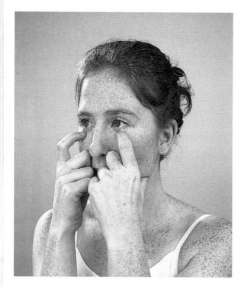

Technique: Rest the thumbs under the jaw-bone and locate the acupoint with the middle or index fingers. Apply acupressure, pressing into the bony socket on both sides.

Benefits: Improves the tone of the skin and muscles on the cheeks and relieves eye problems.

Location: In the depression in front of the notch at the top of the ear. Locate the depression with the mouth open.

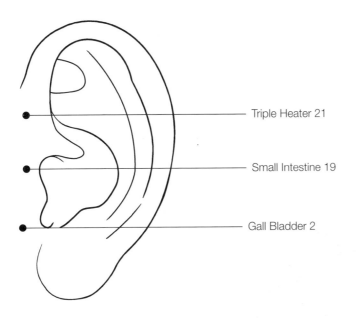

Triple Heater 21

Small Intestine 19

Gall Bladder 2

Technique: Rest the thumbs against the jaw-bone for support and locate the acupoint with the middle or index fingers. Apply acupressure angled slightly upwards towards the top of the ear on both sides.

Benefits: Improves hearing and helps to keep teeth healthy.

12. Small Intestine 19

Location: Just in front of the middle of the ear in the depression formed when the mouth is slightly open.

Technique: Rest the thumbs against the jaw-bone for support and locate the acupoint with the middle or index fingers. Apply acupressure, angled slightly towards the ear, to both sides simultaneously.

Benefits: Improves hearing and can prevent ear infections.

13. Gall Bladder 2

Location: Just behind the jaw-bone and in front of the lobe of the ear, in the depression formed when the mouth is open.

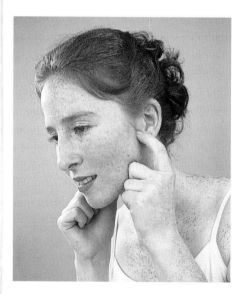

Technique: Rest the thumbs against the jaw-bone for support and locate the acupoint with the middle or index fingers. Apply acupressure perpendicularly behind the top of the jaw-bone.

Benefits: Improves hearing and helps maintain healthy teeth and gums.

14. Stomach 3

Location: On the cheek directly below the pupil of the eye and level with the outside edge of the nostril.

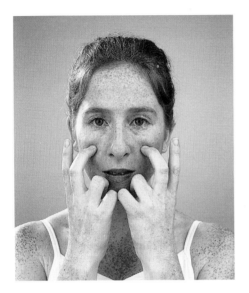

Technique: Rest the thumbs against the jaw-bone for support and locate the acupoint with the middle or index fingers. Apply acupressure perpendicularly, pressing against the cheekbone on both sides.

Benefits: Improves facial skin and helps promote healthy teeth and gums.

15. Large Intestine 20

Location: In the groove in the middle of the outside edge of the nostril.

Technique: Rest the thumbs against the jaw-bone for support and locate the acupoint with the middle or index fingers. Apply acupressure, pressing gently against the bone of the nose on either side.

Benefits: Promotes healthy complexion and clears the nasal passages.

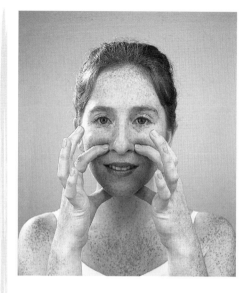

16. Governor Vessel 26

Location: In the groove below the nose, slightly more than halfway up.

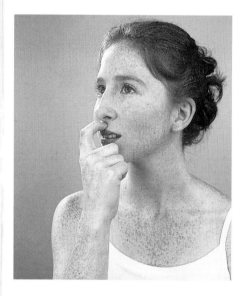

Technique: Locate the point with the nail edge or fingertip of the index or middle finger and place the thumb under the chin for support. Apply acupressure lightly, pressing perpendicularly against the gums underneath.

Caution: Take care not to stimulate this point too hard if you have high blood pressure; stop immediately if you feel unwell or uncomfortable.

Benefits: Tones facial muscles, stimulates gums and improves mental alertness.

17. Stomach 4

Location: At the corner of the mouth, directly below *Acupoint Stomach 3*.

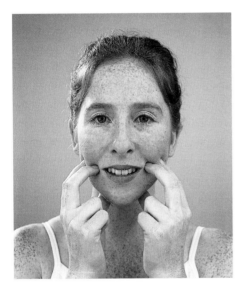

Technique: Rest the thumbs against the jaw-bone for support and locate the acupoint with the middle or index fingers. Apply acupressure, pressing lightly against the teeth and gums underneath on both sides of the mouth.

Benefits: Helps promote oral health and stimulates the skin around the mouth.

18. Stomach 6

Location: Just in front of the lower angle of the jaw-bone, in the depression formed by the muscles when the teeth are clenched.

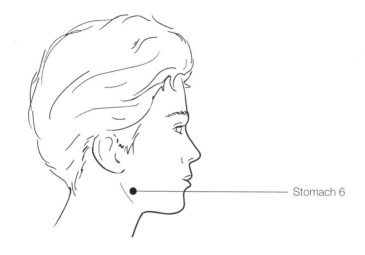

Stomach 6

Technique: Rest the thumbs against the jaw-bone for support and locate the acupoint with the middle or index fingers. Unclench the teeth and apply acupressure, angled slightly upwards, on both sides.

Benefits: Improves the tone of the facial muscles, helps to release tension in the jaw, and promotes saliva and healthy teeth.

19. Conception Vessel 24

Location: In the depression in the centre of the groove of the chin.

Technique: Locate the acupoint with the nail edge or fingertip of the index or middle finger and place the thumb under the chin for support. Apply acupressure, pressing slightly upwards towards the lower lip.

Benefits: Tones the facial muscles and skin, improves the health of the gums and teeth and improves the flow of saliva.

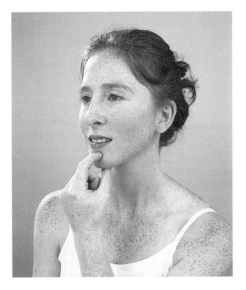

20. Gall Bladder 20

Location: At the back of the head, in the depression between the bottom of the skull and the neck muscles.

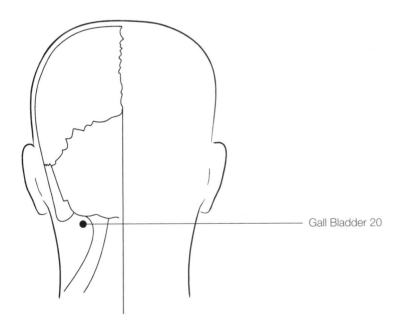

Gall Bladder 20

Technique: Rest the fingers on the back of the head and locate the point with the thumbs. Apply acupressure angled upwards under the edge of the skull on both sides.

Benefits: Releases tension in the head and improves circulation in the face. Also enhances eye function.

Additional Point: Large Intestine 4

Complete the acupressure facial workout by using this vital and potent point, which affects the entire upper body and has an especially beneficial effect on the face and complexion.

Location: In the centre of the triangle made by the bones of the thumb and index finger. Can also be located at the end of the crease made by the index finger and thumb when they are pressed together.

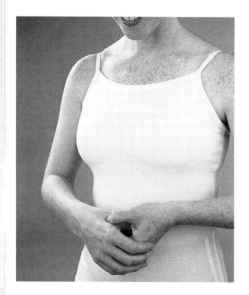

Technique: Support the palm of the left hand in the fingers of the right hand and locate the acupoint with the right thumb. Apply acupressure, angling the thumb slightly towards the wrist.

Note: If pregnant, see pp. 10–11.

Benefits: Improves the complexion, promotes healthy teeth and eyes and clears the nasal passages.

Head and Facial Skin Problems

The facial Acupressure Workout described in the preceding pages will build vitality in the face, improve the complexion and help prevent facial ailments. However, if you suffer from headaches, migraine or acne, the following acupressure points will be of additional benefit.

HEADACHES AND MIGRAINE

Headaches and migraines have a variety of causes. These may include stress, posture, eye problems, spinal problems, hormonal imbalance, constipation, dietary habits, dehydration, allergies or even weather conditions. Keeping a diary of when attacks occur, their severity and what relieves them may help in identifying the main causes. Self-help alongside acupressure can include relaxation exercises, yoga, dietary change and life-style changes. Complementary therapies such as acupuncture, herbal medicine, homoeopathy, osteopathy and massage are also very helpful. For persistent or severe headaches or migraine, seek medical advice.

General acupressure points that will help to prevent and relieve headaches and migraine are as follows:

Governor Vessel 20

Location: At the top of the head on the midline between the tops of the 2 ears and in line with the top of the nose. Locate the point by placing the thumbs on the top of each ear and stretching the middle fingers out to meet at the top of the head.

Technique: Apply acupressure perpendicularly into the scalp, using the middle or index fingertip of one hand. For firmer pressure you can rest the middle or index fingertip of the other hand on top of the nail of the finger locating the point and apply gentle pressure with both fingers simultaneously. The point should be felt as a small depression in the scalp and may feel slightly tender. **Do not overstimulate this point if you have high blood pressure.**

Benefits: Helps to relieve pressure and tension in the head.

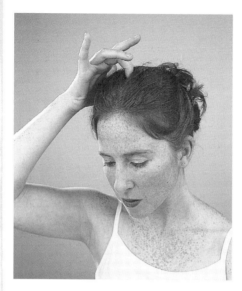

Urinary Bladder 2

Location: On the inner edge of the eyebrow, above the inner corner of each eye.

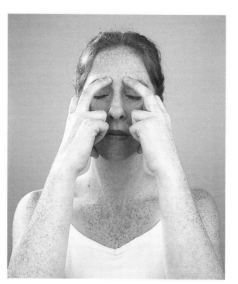

Technique: Locate the acupoint with the thumbs, resting the fingers lightly on the forehead for support or, alternatively, with the index or middle fingers. Apply acupressure with the thumbs or fingers pressing upwards against the bony socket above the eyes.

Benefits: Relieves tension in the forehead and pain around the eyes.

Gall Bladder 1

Location: In the depression level with the outside corner of the eye.

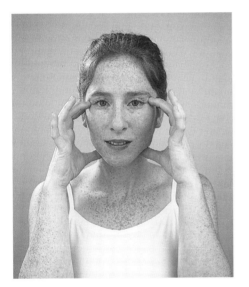

Technique: Resting the thumbs against the jaw-bone for support, locate the acupoint with the index or middle fingers and apply acupressure angled slightly away from the eye on both sides.

Benefits: Relieves headaches and sore eyes.

Gall Bladder 20

Location: At the back of the head, in the depression between the bottom of the skull and the neck muscles.

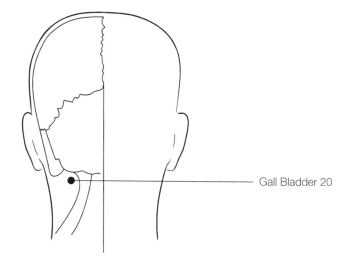

Gall Bladder 20

Technique: Rest the fingers on the back of the head and locate the point with the thumbs. Apply acupressure angled upwards under the edge of the skull on both sides.

Benefits: Relieves headaches and stiff necks.

Large Intestine 4

Location: In the centre of the triangle made by the bones of the thumb and the fingers. Can also be located at the end of the crease made by the index finger and thumb when they are pressed together.

Technique: Support the palm of the left hand in the fingers of the right hand and locate the acupoint with the right thumb. Apply acupressure, angling the thumb slightly towards the wrist. Repeat on the other hand.

Benefits: Relieves headaches and sore eyes.

Note: If pregnant, see pp. 10–11.

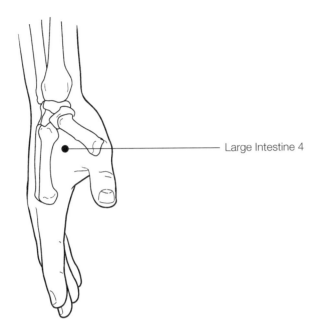

Large Intestine 4

Urinary Bladder 60

Location: In the depression behind the ankle bone on the outside edge of the ankle.

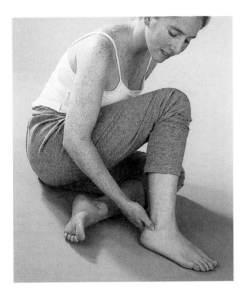

Technique: Place the right hand behind the right leg. Rest the fingers on the inside of the ankle for support and locate the acupoint on the outside edge of the ankle, using the thumb. Apply acupressure with the thumb angled slightly downwards towards the sole of the foot. Alternatively, if it is more comfortable, rest the thumb on the inside ankle and apply pressure with the index or middle finger. Repeat on the other leg.

Benefits: Clears the head, relieves headaches and stiff necks.

Note: If pregnant, see pp. 10–11.

To relieve frontal tension headaches, add the following acupressure points:

Gall Bladder 14

Location: On the forehead about 1 thumb width above the middle of the eyebrows.

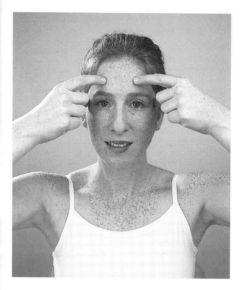

Technique: Place the thumbs against the temples for support and locate the points on both sides of the forehead simultaneously, using the middle or index fingers. Apply acupressure perpendicularly or angled slightly upwards towards the hairline.

Benefits: Relieves frontal headaches and blurred vision.

Location: About 1 finger width inside the hairline on the midline of the scalp in line with the top of the nose.

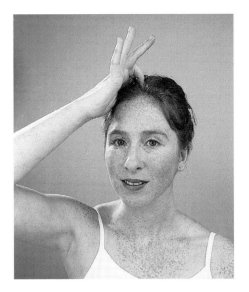

Technique: Apply acupressure perpendicularly, using the middle or index fingertip. Rest the thumb on the temple at the side of the head for support.

Benefits: Relieves frontal headaches and sore eyes.

Forehead Point (Extra Point)

Location: Above the bridge of the nose halfway between the inner edge of each eyebrow.

Technique: Locate with the index or middle fingertip, resting the thumb against the side of the face for support. Apply acupressure angled slightly downwards towards the bridge of the nose.

Benefits: Relieves frontal headaches and forehead pressure due to blocked nose.

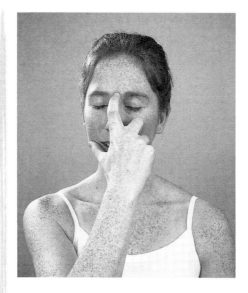

Stomach 36

Location: Four finger widths below the kneecap on the outside edge of the leg bone (tibia).

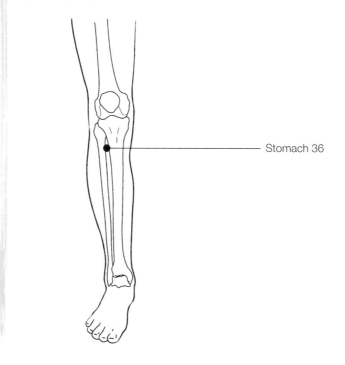

Stomach 36

Technique: Place the fingers behind the leg for support and locate the acupoint with the thumb. Apply acupressure, angled slightly downwards towards the foot, on both legs simultaneously or one at a time.

Benefits: This is an important tonic point for the digestive system and relieves headaches due to digestive imbalance, dietary intolerance or fatigue.

To relieve migraine headaches, add the following acupressure points:

Gall Bladder 1

Location: In the depression level with the outside corner of the eye.

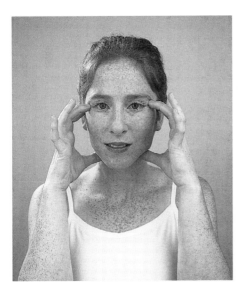

Technique: Resting the thumbs against the jaw-bone for support, locate the acupoint with the index or middle fingers and apply acupressure angled slightly away from the eye on both sides.

Benefits: Relieves one-sided headaches, blurred vision and sore eyes.

Temple Point

Location: In the depression about 1 thumb width behind the midline between the outer edge of the eyebrow and the outer corner of the eye.

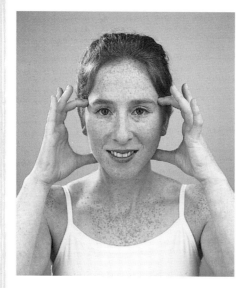

Technique: Rest the thumbs against the jaw-bone for support and locate the point using the index or middle fingers. Apply gentle pressure perpendicularly to both sides.

Benefits: Relieves one-sided headaches and also redness, swelling or soreness of the eyes.

Gall Bladder 8

Location: Within the hairline, 2 finger widths above the top of the ear.

Technique: Resting the thumbs on the jaw-bone for support, locate the top of the ear with the index or middle fingers and then move them about 2 finger widths upwards into the hairline. Apply acupressure to the point, angled slightly towards the back of the head on both sides.

Benefits: Relieves one-sided migraine headaches.

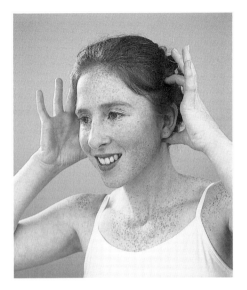

Triple Heater 5

Location: On the outside of the forearm 3 finger widths above the wrist in the depression between the arm bones (radius and ulna).

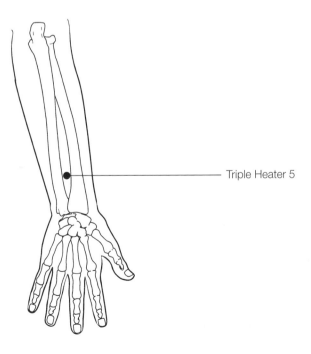

Triple Heater 5

Technique: Measure 3 finger widths from the wrist with the opposite hand. Locate the point with the index finger and support directly underneath the arm with the thumb. Apply acupressure perpendicularly downwards. Repeat on other arm.

Benefits: Relieves migraine and pain in the cheeks.

Gall Bladder 41

Location: On the top of the foot, 3 finger widths above the join between the little and fourth toes, in the depression between the bones.

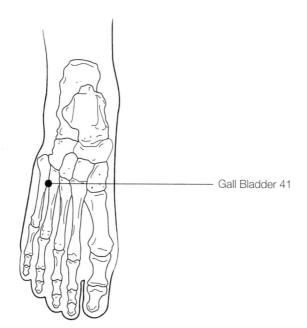

Gall Bladder 41

Technique: Rest fingers under the sole of the foot for support. Locate point with the thumb and apply acupressure angled down towards fourth toe. Repeat on other foot.

Benefits: Relieves migraine, blurred vision and eye pain.

See also The Neck and Shoulders (pp. 114–15), Eye Problems (pp. 86–8) and Sinusitis, Nasal Catarrh and Hay Fever (pp. 96–7).

Acne

Acne may be caused by poor diet, allergies, lack of exercise, stress, environmental pollution or emotional problems. In conjunction with acupressure you could try the following:

- Eat lots of fresh fruit and vegetables, especially leafy greens and foods rich in beta-carotene like carrots, apricots and yellow peppers. Try cutting out dairy products, chocolate and other sugary foods, and all fried and greasy foods. Drink lots of good water and cut down on, or eliminate, coffee and tea. Supplements of zinc may also be helpful.

- Get regular exercise and do daily breathing exercises (outdoors in fresh air is especially beneficial, or else have a window open).

- Learn a relaxation and/or meditation technique to reduce stress and tension.

- Thoroughly cleanse the skin night and morning, and also during the day if it is very greasy. Avoid harsh medicated products and try natural alternatives such as a skin wash made with a few drops of Tea Tree oil in lukewarm water, tepid lime-blossom tea or an infusion of rosemary and sage.

- If emotional problems are also a trigger, find a friend to confide in or consider counselling.

Allergy testing or a nutritional consultation may also be useful (see Useful Addresses section).

Acne may be relieved and prevented by regular use of the following acupoints. Apply acupressure for a few seconds 3 times a day in combination with the general health tips given.

Forehead Point (Extra Point)

Location: Above the bridge of the nose halfway between the inner edge of each eyebrow.

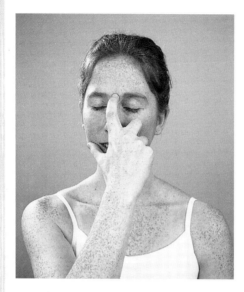

Technique: Locate with the index or middle fingertip, resting the thumb against the side of the face for support. Apply acupressure angled slightly downwards towards the bridge of the nose.

Benefits: Improves facial skin by stimulating the pituitary gland and improving endocrine function in the body.

Stomach 3

Location: On the cheek directly below the pupil of the eye and level with the outside edge of the nostril.

Technique: Rest the thumbs against the jaw-bone for support and locate the acupoint with the middle or index fingers. Apply acupressure perpendicularly, pressing against the cheekbone on both sides.

Benefits: Relieves acne, improves the complexion, promotes healing of facial blemishes.

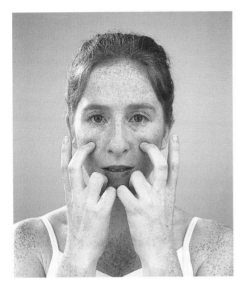

Small Intestine 18

Location: Directly below the outer corner of the eye, just underneath the cheekbone.

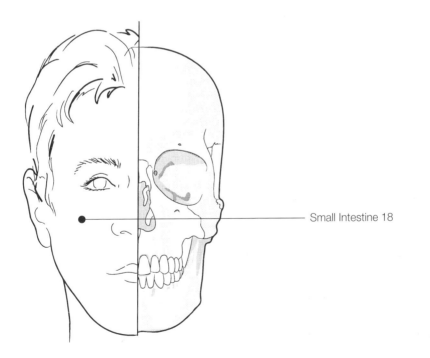

Small Intestine 18

Technique: Rest the thumbs under the jaw-bone for support and locate the point with the middle or index fingers. Apply acupressure angled slightly towards the ears.

Benefits: Improves facial skin by stimulating circulation and aiding digestion.

Gall Bladder 20

Location: At the back of the head, in the depression between the bottom of the skull and the neck muscles.

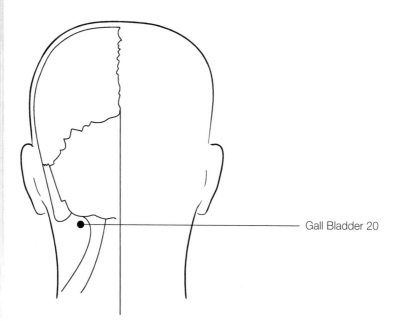

Gall Bladder 20

Technique: Rest the fingers on the back of the head and locate the point with the thumbs. Apply acupressure angled upwards under the edge of the skull on both sides.

Benefits: Relieves tension in the neck, improves circulation to the face.

Location: On the inside edge of the top of the knee, where the opposite thumb touches the muscle when the knee is flexed.

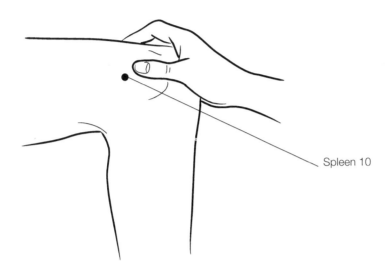

Spleen 10

Technique: Having located the acupoint with the opposite hand, replace it with the same hand, fingers resting on the outside of the knee and thumb applying pressure perpendicularly into the point. Repeat on the other leg.

Benefits: Purifies the blood and improves skin texture and complexion.

Stomach 36

Location: Four finger widths below the kneecap on the outside edge of the leg bone (tibia).

Technique: Place the fingers behind the leg for support and locate the acupoint with the thumb. Apply acupressure angled slightly downwards towards the foot on both legs.

Benefits: Improves digestion and general skin tone; increases vitality.

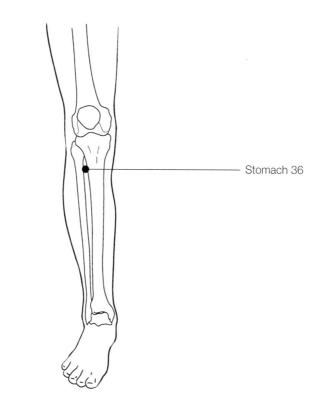

Stomach 36

The Hair

In Oriental medicine healthy hair growth is related to the quality and flow of both blood and vital energy (*chi*) in the body, and also to the general health of the kidneys. So a combination of local points, kidney points, points for toning blood and *chi* is helpful in ensuring luxuriant and glossy hair.

Good diet, adequate sleep and good quality shampoos are also all important for healthy hair. Smoking weakens the hair and it loses lustre. Refined and instant foods also do little for hair appearance, whereas plenty of fresh vegetables, fruit and wholefoods will improve both the hair and complexion. An adequate supply of B vitamins, iron and zinc is also important.

To promote healthy hair growth and improve the condition of your hair, use this acupressure routine twice a week, applying the acupressure to each point for 30 seconds to 1 minute.

Location: At the top of the head on the midline between the tops of the 2 ears and in line with the top of the nose. Locate the point by placing the thumbs on the top of each ear and stretching the middle fingers out to meet at the top of the head.

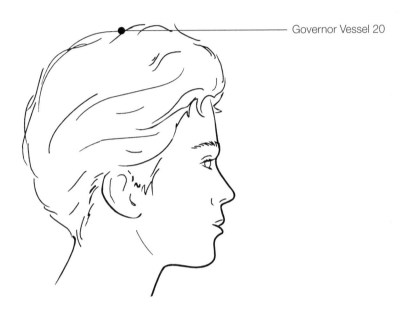

Governor Vessel 20

Technique: Apply acupressure perpendicularly into the scalp, using the middle or index fingertip of one hand. For firmer pressure you can rest the middle or index fingertip of the other hand on top of the nail of the finger locating the point and apply gentle pressure with both fingers simultaneously. The point should be felt as a small depression in the scalp and may feel slightly tender. **Do not overstimulate this point if you have high blood pressure.**

Benefits: Stimulates the scalp and improves local blood flow.

Gall Bladder 8

Location: Within the hairline, 2 finger widths above the top of the ear.

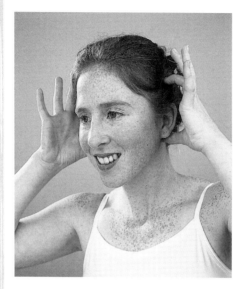

Technique: Resting the thumbs on the jaw-bone for support, locate the top of the ear with the index or middle fingers and then move them about 2 finger widths upwards into the hairline. Apply acupressure to the point, angled slightly towards the back of the head on both sides.

Benefits: Stimulates the flow of blood and *chi* to the scalp. Promotes healthy hair growth.

Gall Bladder 20

Location: At the back of the head, in the depression between the bottom of the skull and the neck muscles.

Technique: Rest the fingers on the back of the head and locate the point with the thumbs. Apply acupressure angled upwards under the edge of the skull on both sides.

Benefits: Reduces stiffness in the neck and improves the circulation of blood and *chi* to the head.

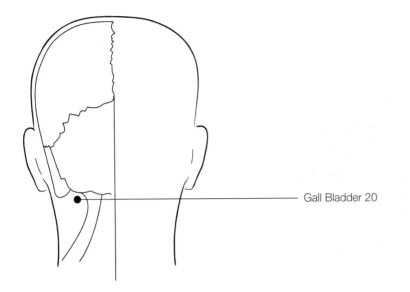

Gall Bladder 20

Triple Heater 5

Location: On the outside of the forearm 3 finger widths above the wrist in the depression between the arm bones (radius and ulna).

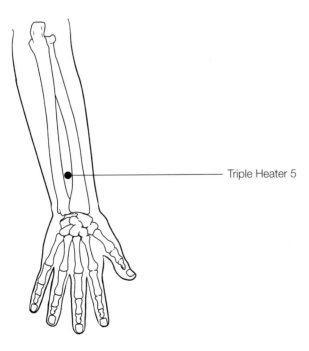

Triple Heater 5

Technique: Measure 3 finger widths from the wrist with the opposite hand. Locate the point with the index finger and support directly underneath the arm with the thumb. Apply acupressure perpendicularly downwards. Repeat on the other arm.

Benefits: An important point that stimulates the flow of blood and *chi* in the head.

Kidney 3

Location: On the inside of the ankle in the depression level with the tip of the ankle bone.

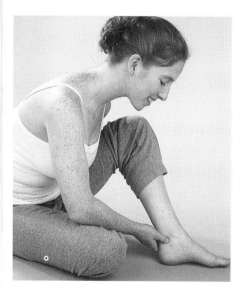

Technique: Place the fingers of the opposite hand behind the ankle for support and locate the point with the thumb. Apply pressure perpendicularly or use small rotations. Repeat on opposite ankle.

Benefits: Stimulates kidney function and promotes healthy hair growth.

DANDRUFF

No-one is sure of the exact cause of dandruff, although diet, stress and fungal infection are all thought to play a part. The above combination of acupressure points used on a daily basis may help. Wash hands thoroughly before and after the acupressure. Also try reducing refined and sugary foods and animal fats in your diet. Cut down on smoking (which dries out the skin) and coffee (which also dehydrates), and increase your intake of cold-pressed plant oils, such as sunflower. Supplements of zinc and B vitamins may help. Avoid harsh anti-dandruff shampoos and try shampoos containing Tea Tree oil, selenium or herbal anti-fungals instead.

BALDNESS

The acupressure points for healthy hair can be used daily to prevent the spread of baldness if it is in the early stages. In the later stages the entire scalp or the area around a patch of baldness should be stimulated daily with a plum-blossom hammer (available from acupuncture supply shops) or a fine-toothed metal comb. Use the plum-blossom hammer (which has 7 small needle tips) or the teeth of the comb to lightly tap over the scalp until it reddens in colour, showing that the flow of blood has increased. Repeat daily, or twice daily if you can manage it, until new hair growth appears. Then continue daily stimulation of the scalp using gentle tapping with the fingertips. Zinc, B and C vitamins, iron and biotin are all thought to be important for hair growth, so make sure you have adequate supplies in your diet or use supplements.

The Eyes

The eyes can be kept healthy and eyesight strengthened both by using local acupoints to increase the flow of blood and *chi* to the eyes and acupoints that stimulate the Liver and Gall Bladder meridians. These 2 meridians are traditionally associated with eye function in Oriental medicine.

You can also maintain healthy eyes by doing regular eye exercises such as yoga exercises or the Bates eye exercises (see Further Reading). Try to get out in the fresh air regularly to allow air to circulate round the eyes and avoid eye-strain due to poor light, neck and facial tension, night driving and too much time spent in front of VDUs, videos and TVs! Plenty of Vitamin A and foods rich in beta-carotene are important too.

Governor Vessel 20

Location: At the top of the head on the midline between the tops of the 2 ears and in line with the top of the nose. Locate the point by placing the thumbs on the top of each ear and stretching the middle fingers out to meet at the top of the head.

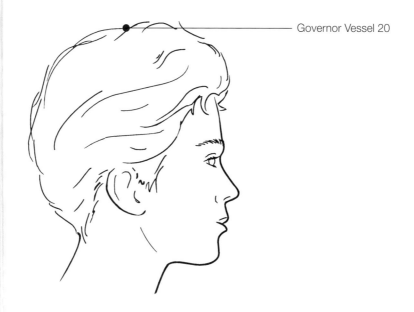

Governor Vessel 20

Technique: Apply acupressure perpendicularly into the scalp, using the middle or index fingertip of one hand. For firmer pressure you can rest the middle or index fingertip of the other hand on top of the nail of the finger locating the point and apply gentle pressure with both fingers simultaneously. The point should be felt as a small depression in the scalp and may feel slightly tender. **Do not overstimulate this point if you have high blood pressure.**

Benefits: Improves circulation to the eyes.

Location: On the inner edge of the eyebrow, above the inner corner of each eye.

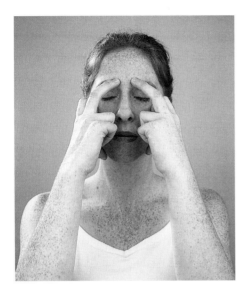

Technique: Locate the acupoint with the thumbs, resting the fingers lightly on the forehead for support or with the index or middle fingers. Apply acupressure with the thumbs or fingers pressing upwards against the bony socket above the eyes.

Benefits: Improves visual ability.

Gall Bladder 1

Location: In the depression level with the outside corner of the eye.

Technique: Resting the thumbs against the jaw-bone for support, locate the acupoint with the index or middle fingers and apply acupressure angled slightly away from the eye on both sides.

Benefits: Strengthens the muscles of the eyes and improves vision.

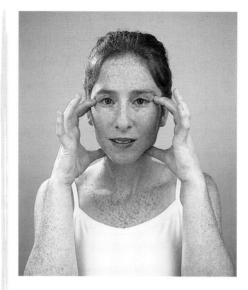

Liver 3

Location: On the top of the foot in the web between the first and second toes, just before the join of the small bones of the foot.

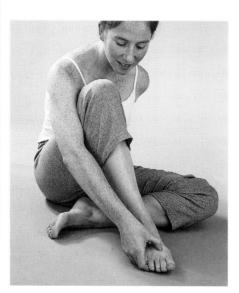

Technique: Place the fingers under the foot for support and press into the point perpendicularly with the thumb. Take care to apply pressure in the hollow between the bone and the tendons rather than on the tendons or blood vessels themselves. Repeat on the other foot.

Benefits: Relieves eye tiredness and increases the flow of *chi* to the eyes.

Gall Bladder 37

Location: On the outside of the leg, about 5 thumb widths above the tip of the ankle bone and just in front of the leg bone (fibula).

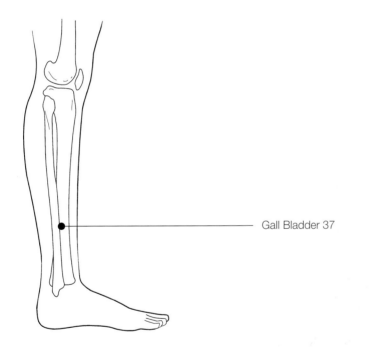

Gall Bladder 37

Technique: Place the fingers behind the ankle and the thumb on the tip of the ankle bone. Measure 5 thumb widths up the leg with the opposite hand. Then slide the thumb up until you locate the sensitive hollow of this acupoint. Apply acupressure angled slightly downwards towards the heel. Repeat on other leg.

Benefits: Brightens the appearance of the eyes.

Eye Problems

EYE-STRAIN

To relieve eye-strain due to tension, use the above acupressure points and add:

Gall Bladder 20

Location: At the back of the head, in the depression between the bottom of the skull and the neck muscles.

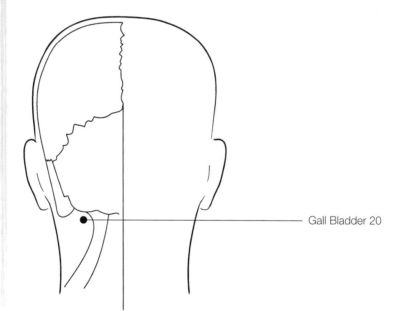

Gall Bladder 20

Technique: Rest the fingers on the back of the head and locate the point with the thumbs. Apply acupressure angled upwards under the edge of the skull on both sides.

Benefits: Relieves neck tension and eases sore or painful eyes.

FAILING EYESIGHT

To improve failing eyesight add:

Gall Bladder 1

Location: In the depression level with the outside corner of the eye.

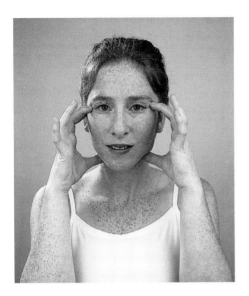

Technique: Resting the thumbs against the jaw-bone for support, locate the acupoint with the index or middle fingers and apply acupressure angled slightly away from the eye on both sides.

Benefits: Improves failing eyesight and eases sore eyes.

EYE TWITCHING

To reduce eye twitching add:

Gall Bladder 14

Location: On the forehead about 1 thumb width above the middle of the eyebrows.

Technique: Place the thumbs against the temples for support and locate the points on both sides of the forehead simultaneously, using the middle or index fingers. Apply acupressure angling slightly upwards towards the hairline.

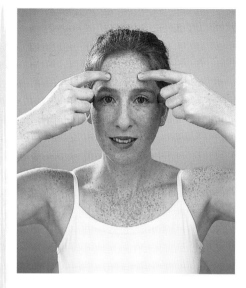

Benefits: Reduces twitching of the eyelids and improves blurred vision.

WATERY EYES

To treat eyes that water easily, add the above point (*Gall Bladder 14*) and:

Gall Bladder 15

Location: Directly above the midpoint of the eyebrows, 1 finger width within the hairline.

Technique: Place the thumbs on the temples for support and locate the point using the index or middle fingers of each hand. Apply pressure perpendicularly against the skull on both sides.

Benefits: Reduces eye watering, especially on exposure to wind, and improves blurred vision.

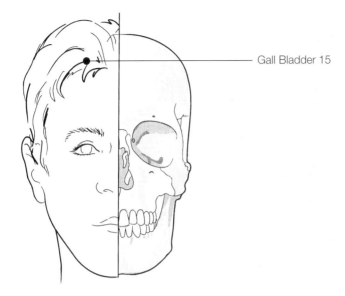

Gall Bladder 15

The Ears

Good hearing can be promoted by using local ear points and a tonic point on the Kidney meridian, traditionally associated with hearing ability. If you are a frequent swimmer, water-borne ear infections can be prevented by wearing ear plugs that keep the inside of the ear dry. There are also a number of Chinese *Qi gong* exercises to strengthen hearing and prevent deafness (see Further Reading).

Persistent hearing impairment or ear pain should be checked medically as it may indicate disease, infection or damage to the ear bones.

Triple Heater 21

Location: In the depression in front of the notch at the top of the ear. Locate the depression with the mouth open.

Technique: Rest the thumbs against the jaw-bone for support and locate the acupoint with the middle or index fingers. Apply acupressure angled slightly upwards towards the top of the ear on both sides.

Benefits: Improves hearing.

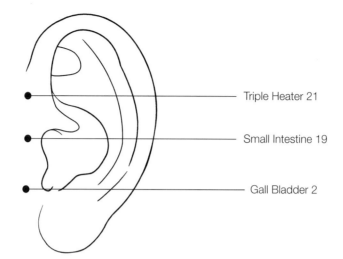

Triple Heater 21

Small Intestine 19

Gall Bladder 2

Small Intestine 19

Location: Just in front of the middle of the ear in the depression formed when the mouth is slightly open.

Technique: Rest the thumbs against the jaw-bone for support and locate the acupoint with the middle or index fingers. Apply acupressure angled slightly towards the ear on both sides.

Benefits: Improves hearing.

Gall Bladder 2

Location: Just behind the jaw-bone and in front of the lobe of the ear, in the depression formed when the mouth is open.

Technique: Rest the thumbs against the jaw-bone for support and locate the acupoint with the middle or index fingers. Apply acupressure perpendicularly behind the top of the jaw-bone on both sides.

Benefits: Improves hearing.

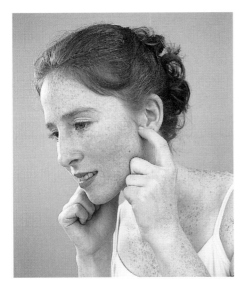

Kidney 3

Location: On the inside of the ankle in the depression level with the tip of the ankle bone.

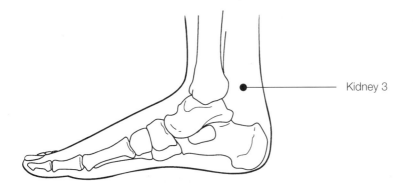

Kidney 3

Technique: Place the fingers of the opposite hand behind the ankle for support and locate the point with the thumb. Apply pressure perpendicularly or use small rotations. Repeat on the opposite ankle.

Benefits: Strengthens hearing ability.

Ear Problems

DEAFNESS, RINGING IN THE EARS (TINNITUS) AND EAR INFECTIONS

The ear points given above will all help to prevent and relieve deafness, ringing in the ears and ear infections.

For severe hearing impairment add:

Urinary Bladder 23

Location: On the lower back 2 finger widths on either side of the spine, approximately level with the waist, by the lower edge of the second lumbar vertebra.

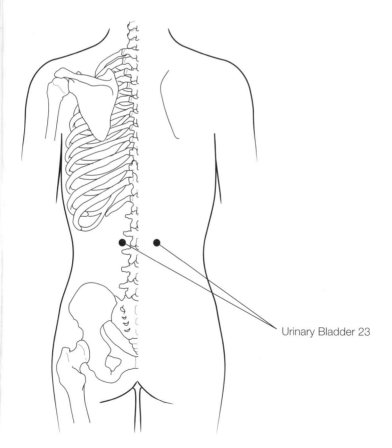

Urinary Bladder 23

Technique: Place the thumbs on either side of the waist and locate the point on both sides of the spine using the middle fingers. Alternatively, lie on the floor and, arching the back slightly, place the knuckles or two tennis balls level with the points and then gently lower the back onto them.

Benefits: Stimulates ear function and reduces tinnitus.

The Nose

To promote a good sense of smell and prevent nasal irritations and blockage, the following acupressure points are excellent:

Governor Vessel 20

Location: At the top of the head on the midline between the tops of the 2 ears and in line with the top of the nose. Locate the point by placing the thumbs on the top of each ear and stretching the middle fingers out to meet at the top of the head.

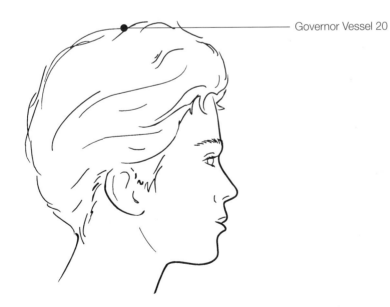

Governor Vessel 20

Technique: Apply acupressure perpendicularly into the scalp, using the middle or index fingertip of one hand. For firmer pressure you can rest the middle or index fingertip of the other hand on top of the nail of the finger locating the point and apply gentle pressure with both fingers simultaneously. The point should be felt as a small depression in the scalp and may feel slightly tender. **Do not overstimulate this point if you have high blood pressure.**

Benefits: Helps clear the nasal passages.

Large Intestine 20

Location: In the groove in the middle of the outside edge of the nostril.

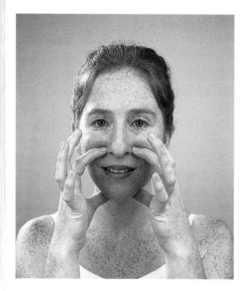

Technique: Rest the thumbs against the jaw-bone for support and locate the acupoint with the middle or index fingers. Apply acupressure, pressing gently against the bone of the nose on both sides.

Benefits: Clears nasal obstructions and heightens the sense of smell.

Large Intestine 4

Location: In the centre of the triangle made by the bones of the thumb and the fingers. Can also be located at the end of the crease made by the index finger and thumb when they are pressed together.

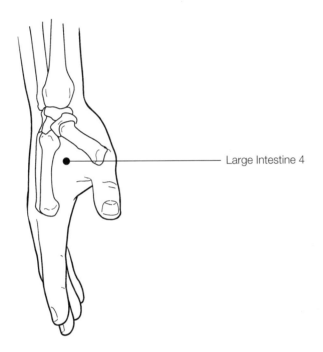

Large Intestine 4

Technique: Support the palm of the left hand in the fingers of the right hand and locate the acupoint with the right thumb. Apply acupressure, angling the thumb slightly towards the wrist. Repeat on opposite hand.

Benefits: Stimulates the flow of energy in the upper body and clears the nose.

Note: If pregnant, see pp. 10–11.

Nasal Problems

The above points can also help prevent and relieve common nasal problems.

LOSS OF SENSE OF SMELL

This is an increasingly common problem. Regular use of the above points, combined with breathing exercises, and zinc supplementation may help.

SINUSITIS, NASAL CATARRH AND HAY FEVER

To relieve sinusitis, a build up of nasal catarrh or hay fever, use the above points 2–3 times daily until relief is obtained. Cut out dairy products and cold foods and drinks, which are mucus-producing, until symptoms subside. Also avoid constipation, which can contribute to nasal blockage. You may also add the following points:

Urinary Bladder 2

Location: On the inner edge of the eyebrow, above the inner corner of each eye.

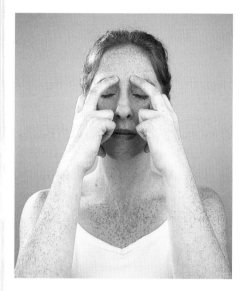

Technique: Locate the acupoint with the thumbs, resting the fingers lightly on the forehead for support or with the middle or index fingers. Apply acupressure with the thumbs pressing upwards against the bony socket above the eyes.

Benefits: Helps to clear the sinuses.

acupressure

simple steps

to health

Location: On the nape of the neck, just inside the hairline, 2 finger widths on either side of the spine in the depression on the side of the large neck muscle (trapezius).

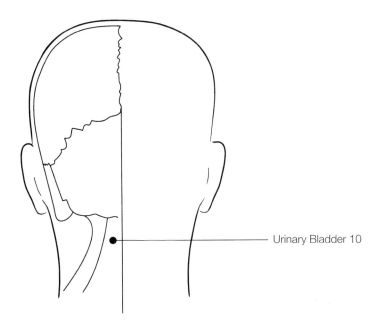

Urinary Bladder 10

Technique: Rest the fingers on the back of the scalp. Locate the acupoint with the thumbs and apply pressure perpendicularly to the base of the skull on both sides.

Benefits: Clears the head and the nasal passages. Relieves sinusitis.

NOSEBLEEDS

To prevent, or stop, nosebleeds, use the above points and add:

Stomach 3

Location: On the cheek directly below the pupil of the eye and level with the outside edge of the nostril.

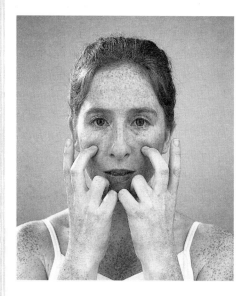

Technique: Rest the thumbs against the jaw-bone for support and locate the acupoint with the middle or index fingers. Apply acupressure perpendicularly, pressing against the cheekbone on both sides.

Benefits: First aid point for a nosebleed. Regular use will also help prevent nosebleeds.

To stop a nosebleed, sit down with the head well forward, loosening clothing and breathing through the mouth. Pinch the soft part of the base of the nose and apply acupressure to the points given above. If you have someone to help you, let them apply the acupressure while you hold the nose or vice versa. *Don't* raise your head or plug the nose and try not to blow the nose for a few hours after the bleeding has stopped. Frequent nosebleeds may be a sign of tension or blood pressure problems. If regular use of these acupressure points does not reduce nosebleeds, you should consult your doctor for a check-up.

The points listed under the common cold (pp. 137–9) may also help relieve and prevent general nasal problems.

The Mouth

Acupressure can help promote healthy teeth and gums and prevent mouth and throat problems.

To promote oral health and sweet-smelling breath, take care of your diet and cut down on sweet, sticky foods. Pay scrupulous attention to dental hygiene, including regular, careful brushing and flossing. Massage the gums gently with the fingertips and stimulate saliva by massaging the gums with the tongue while the mouth is closed. Herbal mouthwashes with a few drops of lavender or Tea Tree oil are gentler than antiseptic mouthwashes but just as effective.

General acupoints for oral health are:

Large Intestine 4

Location: In the centre of the triangle made by the bones of the thumb and the fingers. Can also be located at the end of the crease made by the index finger and thumb when they are pressed together.

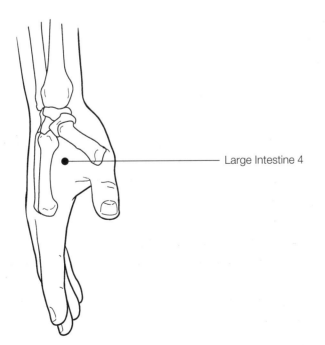

Large Intestine 4

Technique: Support the palm of the left hand in the fingers of the right hand and locate the acupoint with the right thumb. Apply acupressure, angling the thumb slightly towards the wrist. Repeat on opposite hand.

Benefits: Promotes oral hygiene and strengthens the teeth.

Note: If pregnant, see pp. 10–11.

Stomach 4

Location: At the corner of the mouth, directly below *Acupoint Stomach 3*.

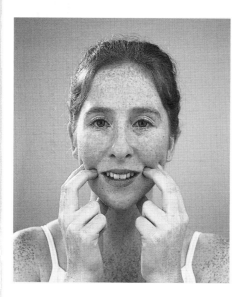

Technique: Rest the thumbs against the jaw-bone for support and locate the acupoint with the middle or index fingers. Apply acupressure, pressing lightly against the teeth and gums underneath, on both sides of the mouth.

Benefits: Stimulates healthy saliva production and improves oral health.

Location: Four finger widths below the kneecap on the outside edge of the leg bone (tibia).

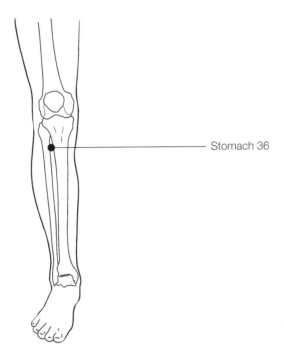

Stomach 36

Technique: Place the fingers behind the leg for support and locate the acupoint with the thumb. Apply acupressure angled slightly downwards towards the foot. Repeat on opposite leg.

Benefits: Aids digestion, helps to sweeten the breath.

Mouth Problems

MOUTH ULCERS AND MOUTH IRRITATION

Ulcers are often a sign of stress or feeling run down; they are more common in women around the time of their periods. They can be prevented by regular intake of vitamins B and C in foods or supplements. Relief may also be obtained by dabbing the ulcer with a freshly cut clove of garlic.

To relieve mouth ulcers and mouth irritation, use the above acupoints every few hours at the first signs of discomfort and add:

Urinary Bladder 10

Location: On the nape of the neck, just inside the hairline, 2 finger widths on either side of the spine in the depression on the side of the large neck muscle (trapezius).

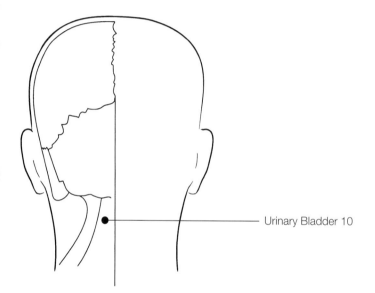

Urinary Bladder 10

Technique: Rest the fingers on the back of the scalp. Locate the acupoint with the thumbs and apply pressure perpendicularly to the base of the skull on either side.

Benefits: Relieves tension and discomfort in the mouth.

TOOTHACHE AND DENTAL PROBLEMS

Acupressure can ease toothache, minimize the need for dental anaesthesia and also help relieve pain during and after dental treatment. For toothache, use the general oral points every few hours. During dental treatment, *Large Intestine 4* (see above) can be pressed constantly to alleviate discomfort. Stimulate the acupoint on the hand *opposite* the affected side of the mouth. The following additional points may also be useful for toothache or pain after dental treatment.

Stomach 6

Location: Just in front of the lower angle of the jaw-bone, in the depression formed by the muscles when the teeth are clenched.

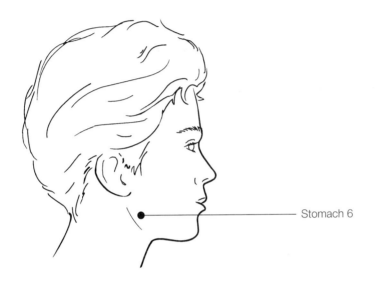

Stomach 6

Technique: Rest the thumbs against the jaw-bone for support and locate the acupoint with the middle or index fingers. Unclench the teeth and apply acupressure angled slightly upwards on both sides.

Benefits: Relieves toothache and swelling in the face.

Stomach 7

Location: At the side of the cheek in the depression under the cheekbone in front of the ear lobe.

Technique: Rest thumbs under the jaw and locate acupoint with middle or index fingers, applying acupressure angled slightly upwards under cheekbone on both sides.

Benefits: Relieves toothache, swelling and facial pain.

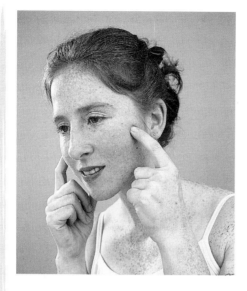

Large Intestine 11

Location: In the depression at the end of the elbow crease, when the elbow is bent.

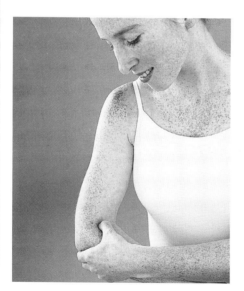

Technique: Support the elbow in the fingers and palm of the opposite hand and locate the point with the thumb. Apply acupressure angled slightly towards the elbow and upper arm. Repeat on the opposite arm.

Benefits: Relieves toothache and pain in the mouth.

SORE THROATS, LARYNGITIS AND TONSILLITIS

Sore throats may be due to stress and being run down, dry air and air pollutants, infections or voice strain. Take plenty of fluids and increase humidity in the air. Increase your intake of vitamin C and add garlic to your food. Get plenty of rest and gargle with a mild antiseptic or herbal preparation such as red sage tea and honey (avoid sage if you are pregnant). If you often strain your voice when speaking or singing, get training on how to use it properly. Regular acupressure will prevent recurrent throat infections. In Oriental medicine the throat is related to the kidney meridian so stimulating points for the kidneys (see Chapter 7, The Urinary System, pp. 177–88) is also beneficial.

To relieve sore throats, laryngitis and tonsillitis, use the general mouth points every few hours and add:

Gall Bladder 20

Location: At the back of the head, in the depression between the bottom of the skull and the neck muscles.

Technique: Rest fingers on the back of the head and locate the point with the thumbs. Apply acupressure angled upwards under the edge of the skull on both sides.

Benefits: Relieves neck and shoulder tension and eases sore throats.

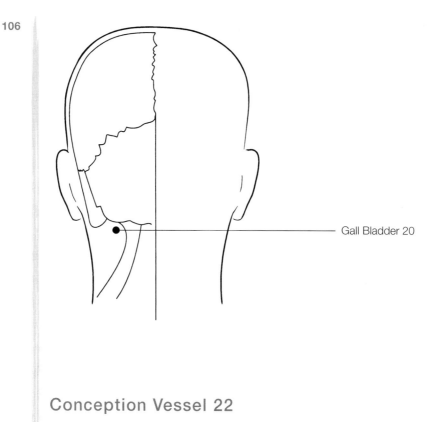

Gall Bladder 20

Conception Vessel 22

Location: In the depression below the throat, just above the top of the breastbone.

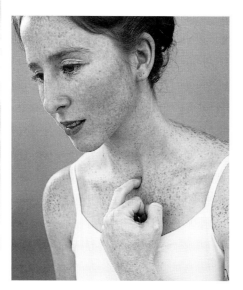

Technique: Locate the point with the middle or index finger and press in against the bone, not against the windpipe.

Benefits: Relieves sore throat and voice hoarseness.

Lung 5

Location: On the inside of the elbow in the hollow on the outer edge of the tendons when the elbow is slightly bent.

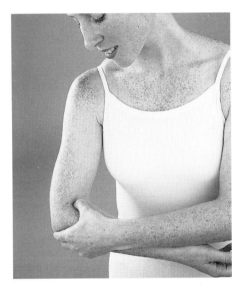

Technique: Support the elbow in the fingers of the opposite hand and locate the acupoint with the thumb. Apply acupressure perpendicularly and repeat on opposite arm.

Benefits: Relieves sore throat and strengthens the voice.

| Urinary Bladder 23

Location: On the lower back 2 finger widths on either side of the spine, approximately level with the waist, by the lower edge of the second lumbar vertebra.

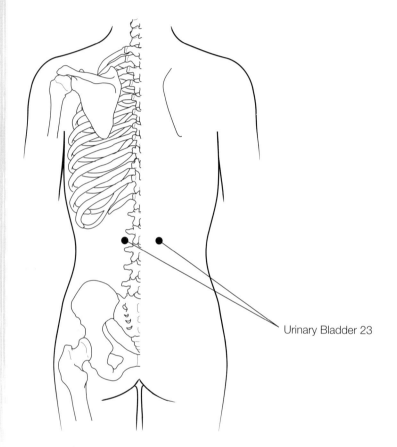

Urinary Bladder 23

Technique: Place the thumbs on either side of the waist and locate the point on both sides of the spine using the middle fingers. Alternatively, lie on the floor and, arching the back slightly, place the knuckles or two tennis balls level with the points and then gently lower the back onto them.

Benefits: Stimulates kidney function, relieves tiredness and eases sore throats.

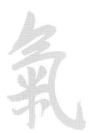

Healthy Joints

Certain acupoints help to strengthen the joints and stimulate bone formation generally. Others influence specific joints or help to strengthen the muscles that support the joints. Use the acupoints described below (3 of which are included in the Acupressure Workout) on a daily basis to build strength in the joints and bones and prevent injury. You can also add other specific acupoints for particular joints that are weak, prone to injury or damaged.

Regular weight-bearing exercise helps to build up bone and strengthen the joints and their surrounding muscles and tendons, while massage and meridian stretches (see Further Reading) can help to loosen stiff joints. Make sure that you consume plenty of calcium, magnesium and essential fatty acids in your diet and decrease your intake of sugary and acidic foods.

Urinary Bladder 11

Location: At the back of the neck in line with the shoulders and level with the lower edge of the first thoracic vertebra. Located 2 finger widths on either side of the spine.

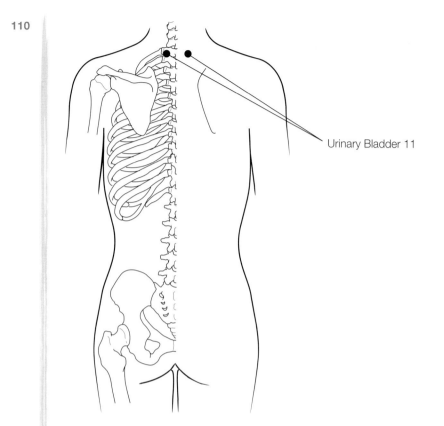

Urinary Bladder 11

Technique: Reach the hands over the back of the neck and locate the point with the index or middle fingers. Apply firm pressure perpendicularly on either side of the spine.

Benefits: The most influential point for bone in the body; helps to promote strong, healthy bones and joints throughout the body.

Urinary Bladder 40

Location: At the back of the knee, between the tendons.

Technique: Bend the knees slightly and place the thumbs at the side of the kneecaps for support and the fingers behind the knees. Locate the point with the index or middle fingers, feeling gently for the hollow in between the tendons. Do not press on the tendons themselves and avoid any varicose veins.

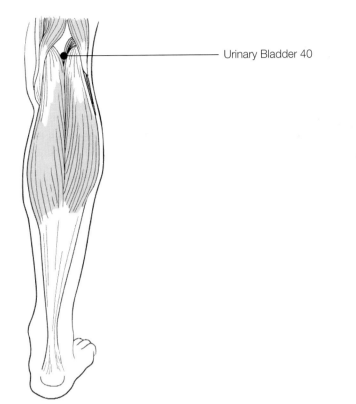

Urinary Bladder 40

Benefits: Strengthens the joints in the lower body, especially the lower back, hips and knees.

Gall Bladder 39

Location: On the outside of the leg 4 finger widths above the tip of the ankle bone in the depression between the bone and the tendons.

Technique: Place the fingers behind the leg for support and locate the point with the thumb. Apply acupressure angled slightly downwards towards the heel. Repeat on opposite leg.

Benefits: This point strengthens the bones throughout the body, particularly the knee and ankle joints.

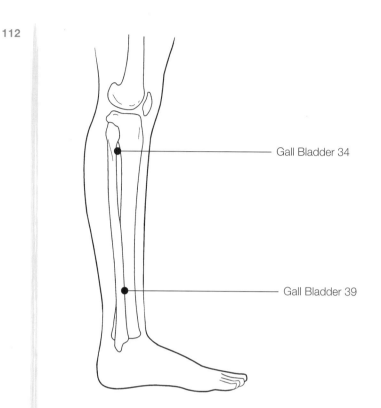

Gall Bladder 34

Gall Bladder 39

Gall Bladder 34

Location: On the outside of the leg in the hollow just beneath the meeting point of the 2 leg bones, approximately 1 thumb width above and 2 finger widths to the outside of acupoint *Stomach 36*.

Technique: Place the fingers round the outsides of the legs, just below the knees, and locate the point using the thumbs. Apply pressure angled down towards the feet.

Benefits: This point strengthens the tendons and muscles that support the joints throughout the body. It is particularly helpful for knee joint pain or motor impairment of the leg.

Acupoints to Strengthen or Treat Specific Joints

Select from the acupoints below as appropriate and add them to the sequence of points described above.

To relieve a stiff and aching jaw, often caused by unconscious grinding of the teeth during sleep, add the following point. Facial massage or self-massage of the jaw may also help to release tension. Try to be aware of the build up of tension in the jaw during the day and loosen it by applying acupressure to this point and gently shaking the jaw loose. It is also useful to apply acupressure to this point just before sleeping.

Stomach 6

Location: Just in front of the lower angle of the jaw-bone, in the depression formed by the muscles when the teeth are clenched.

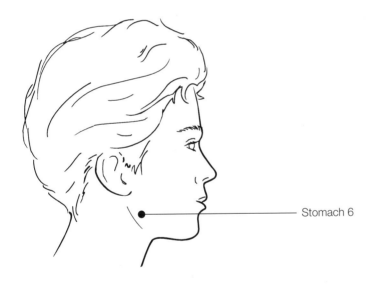

Stomach 6

Technique: Rest the thumbs against the jaw-bone for support and locate the acupoint with the middle or index fingers. Unclench the teeth and apply acupressure angled slightly upwards on both sides of the face.

Benefits: Relieves pain and stiffness in the jaw and releases spasm of the jaw muscles.

THE NECK AND SHOULDERS

Neck and shoulder stiffness and pain may be due to poor posture, uncomfortable pillows or bed, poor circulation or tension and anxiety. Massage can be combined well with acupressure to relieve tension. Posture, especially when sitting at desks and working on VDUs, should be checked. Some people get relief from orthopaedic pillows. Deep breathing and relaxation techniques may help.

To relieve stiffness and tension in the neck and shoulders, add the following points:

Gall Bladder 20

Location: At the back of the head, in the depression between the bottom of the skull and the neck muscles.

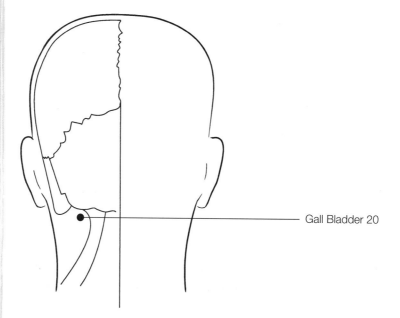

Gall Bladder 20

Technique: Rest the fingers on the back of the head and locate the point with the thumbs. Apply acupressure angled upwards under the edge of the skull on both sides of the spine.

Benefits: Releases pain and stiffness of the neck, shoulder and upper back.

Location: Halfway between the highest point of the shoulder and the junction between the last vertebrae of the neck and the first vertebrae of the upper back.

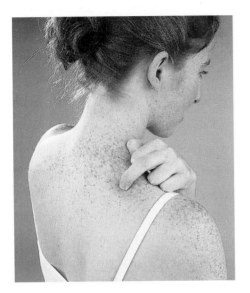

Technique: Place one hand over the opposite shoulder and locate the point using the middle or index finger. Apply acupressure angled slightly downwards. Repeat on opposite side.

Benefits: Eases stiffness in the neck and relieves pain in the shoulder and back.

THE ELBOWS

The elbow joint can be damaged by rapid jerking, sports injuries or falls. Warm up the joint before exercise and wear a support bandage if the joint is uncomfortable. Add the following points to relieve elbow stiffness and pain:

Large Intestine 11

Location: In the depression at the end of the elbow crease, when the elbow is bent.

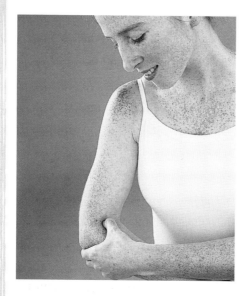

Technique: Support the elbow in the fingers and palm of the opposite hand and locate the point with the thumb. Apply acupressure angled slightly towards the elbow and upper arm. Repeat on opposite arm.

Benefits: Relieves pain and increases mobility of the elbow and arm.

Triple Heater 5

Location: On the outside of the forearm 3 finger widths above the wrist in the depression between the arm bones (radius and ulna).

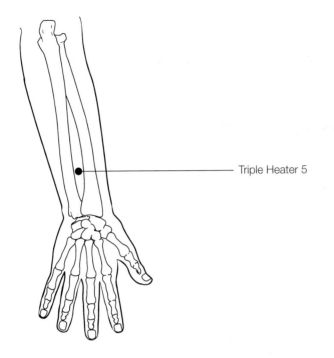

Triple Heater 5

Technique: Measure 3 finger widths from the wrist with the opposite hand. Locate the point with the index finger and support directly underneath the arm with the thumb. Apply acupressure perpendicularly downwards. Repeat on other arm.

Benefits: Increases mobility of the elbow and relieves pain in the arm and fingers.

THE WRISTS

The wrists can be strained or sprained during daily activities or sport. Keyboard operators with poor posture are especially liable to wrist strain, as are participants in racquet sports. Pregnant and middle-aged women can be prone to Carpal Tunnel Syndrome, involving pain, numbness and tingling in the wrist. These conditions may be relieved by acupressure to the following points.

Regular release of wrist tension during daily activities, and the inclusion of wrist and finger exercises, will help prevent and ease wrist problems. For example, keyboard operators should stop typing for a few minutes every hour, shake out the hands, rotate the wrists gently and stretch the fingers. The use of wrist supports and support bandages can also help.

Triple Heater 5

Location: See previous page.

Technique: See previous page.

Benefits: Relieves pain and increases circulation in the wrist and fingers.

Pericardium 6

Location: Between the tendons on the inside of the arm, 3 finger widths above the wrist crease closest to the palm.

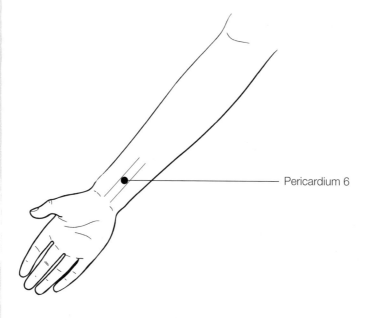

Pericardium 6

Technique: Measure up from the wrist crease to locate the point. Support the wrist with the fingers of the opposite hand and apply acupressure to the point using the thumb, angled downwards towards the middle finger. Repeat on other wrist.

Benefits: Relieves pain in the elbow and wrist and relaxes muscles in the arm.

Unconscious tension may be stored in the hands and fingers during daily activities, for example when writing, carrying shopping or holding objects. This can be relieved by resting the hands at regular intervals and including finger exercises in the daily routine. The following additional acupressure points are also helpful:

Large Intestine 4

Location: In the centre of the triangle made by the bones of the thumb and the fingers. Can also be located at the end of the crease made by the index finger and thumb when they are pressed together.

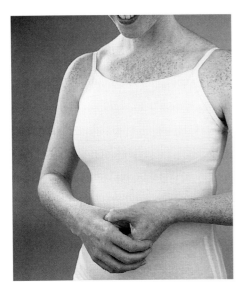

Technique: Support the palm of the left hand in the fingers of the right hand and locate the acupoint with the right thumb. Apply acupressure, angling the thumb slightly towards the wrist.

Benefits: Releases tension and pain in the hands and fingers.

Note: If pregnant, see pp. 10–11.

| # Triple Heater 4

Location: On the wrist in the depression between the bones when the wrist is flexed slightly upwards, in line with the ring finger.

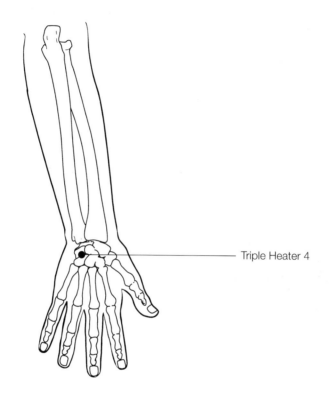

Triple Heater 4

Technique: Support the wrist with the fingers of the opposite hand and locate the point with the thumb. Apply acupressure angled slightly upwards towards the elbow. Repeat on opposite arm.

Benefits: Relieves pain in the wrists, hands and fingers.

THE BACK

To maintain a healthy back, regular gentle exercise of the spine is important (meridian or yoga stretches are ideal – see Further Reading section) especially first thing in the morning. Many back injuries occur during the first hour after waking. Posture is also crucial when working, walking, sitting and sleeping. Posture can be improved, and backache markedly relieved, with therapies such as the Alexander Technique, Feldenkreis, Pilates or other bodywork techniques. Some relief may also be obtained using support or orthopaedic cushions and pillows. For severe or chronic problems, osteopathy cranio-sacral therapy or chiropractic treatment are helpful. Back problems can also be related to weak bladder or kidney function so improving these can be beneficial (see Chapter 7, The Urinary System, pp. 177–88).

For pain in the upper back, add the following acupoints:

Gall Bladder 21

Location: Halfway between the highest point of the shoulder and the junction between the last vertebrae of the neck and the first vertebrae of the upper back.

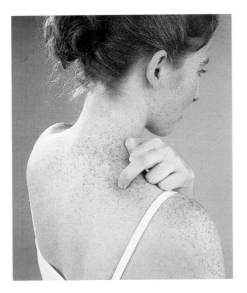

Technique: Place one hand over the opposite shoulder and locate the point using the middle or index finger. Apply acupressure angled slightly downwards. Repeat on other side.

Benefits: Relieves pain in the upper back and shoulders.

Large Intestine 11

Location: In the depression at the end of the elbow crease, when the elbow is bent.

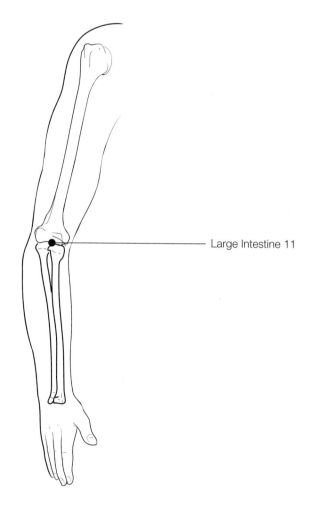

Large Intestine 11

Technique: Support the elbow in the fingers and palm of the opposite hand and locate the point with the thumb. Apply acupressure angled slightly towards the elbow and upper arm. Repeat on other arm.

Benefits: Relieves stiffness and pain in the upper body.

For relief of pain and stiffness in the middle of the back, add the following:

Urinary Bladder 18

Location: Two finger widths on either side of the spine, level with the ninth thoracic vertebra.

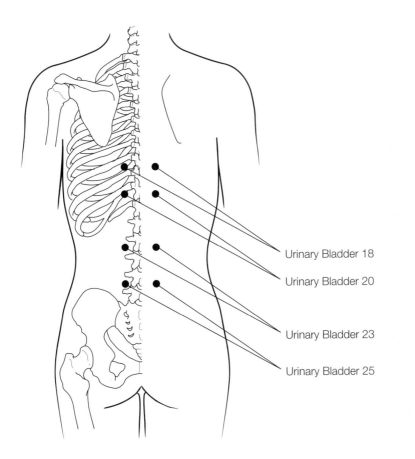

Urinary Bladder 18

Urinary Bladder 20

Urinary Bladder 23

Urinary Bladder 25

Technique: Lie on the floor with the knees bent and place either the knuckles or two tennis balls under the back level with the point. Gradually lower the weight of the back onto the knuckles or balls to apply acupressure to the point on both sides of the spine.

Benefits: Relieves pain in the middle of the back and around the ribs.

Urinary Bladder 20

Location: Two finger widths on either side of the spine, level with the eleventh thoracic vertebra.

Technique: As for *Urinary Bladder 18* (previous page).

Benefits: Relieves pain in the middle of the back and upper abdomen.

To relieve sciatica and pain and stiffness in the lower back, add the following points:

Urinary Bladder 23

Location: On the lower back 2 finger widths on either side of the spine, approximately level with the waist, by the lower edge of the second lumbar vertebra.

Technique: Place the thumbs on either side of the waist and locate the point on both sides of the spine using the middle fingers. Alternatively, lie on the floor and, arching the back slightly, place two tennis balls level with the points and then gently lower the back onto them.

Benefits: Relieves pain and weakness in the lower back.

Urinary Bladder 25

Location: Two finger widths on either side of the spine, level with the fourth lumbar vertebra and crest of the hipbones.

Technique: Place the thumbs around the hips and locate the point with the middle fingers, applying acupressure deep into the tissue on either side of the spine.

Alternatively, lie on the floor and apply pressure using the knuckles or tennis balls as for *Urinary Bladder 18* and *20*.

Benefits: Relieves low back pain and constipation.

Urinary Bladder 40

Location: At the back of the knee, between the tendons.

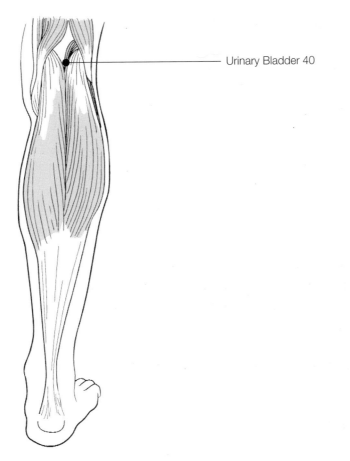

Urinary Bladder 40

Technique: Bend the knees slightly and place the thumbs at the side of the kneecaps for support and the fingers behind the knees. Locate the point with the index or middle fingers, feeling gently for the hollow in between the tendons. Do not press on the tendons themselves and avoid any varicose veins.

Benefits: Relieves pain in the lower back and legs.

Urinary Bladder 60

Location: In the depression behind the ankle bone on the outside edge of the ankle.

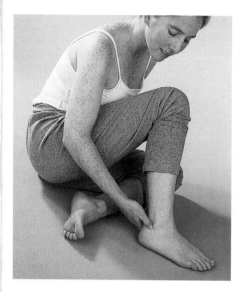

Technique: Place the right hand behind the right leg. Rest the fingers on the inside of the ankle for support and locate the acupoint on the outside edge of the ankle, using the thumb. Apply acupressure with the thumb angled slightly downwards towards the sole of the foot. Alternatively, if it is more comfortable, rest the thumb on the inside ankle and apply pressure with the index or middle finger. Repeat on opposite ankle.

Benefits: Relieves pain in the lower back, legs and heels.

Note: If pregnant, see pp. 10–11.

THE HIPS

Hip mobility can be maintained by daily gentle hip rotations, regular walking and avoiding being seated for long periods without movement. Good posture and pelvic alignment are also important. Osteopathic treatment and orthotics in shoes can balance the pelvis and prevent uneven strain in one hip. To relieve hip pain, add the following:

Location: On the side of the buttock in the depression underneath the thigh bone and two thirds of the distance between the tip of the sacrum and the crest of the hip.

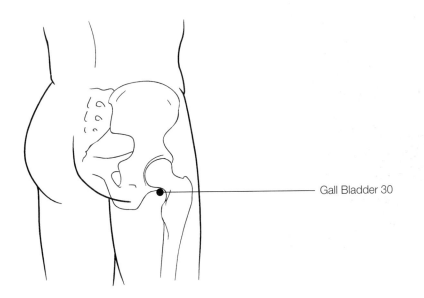

Gall Bladder 30

Technique: Locate this point lying on your side with the thigh raised. Press into the point firmly with either the middle or index finger or the knuckle. Roll over onto the other side and repeat.

Benefits: Relieves pain and increases mobility in the hip and lower back.

THE KNEES

The knee joints can be strengthened with regular, gentle exercise involving stretching and flexing the legs and bending the knees. Avoid straining the knees and do not overburden them with excess body weight. If weight-bearing exercise is painful, try swimming instead. Herbal compresses or hot packs may also be helpful unless the knee is inflamed or swollen, in which case ice packs will be more comfortable. Stimulating the kidney and bladder meridians can help too (see Urinary Health, pp. 177–88).

To relieve stiffness and pain in the knees, add the following acupoints:

Knee Acupoints

Location: In the depressions just above and below the kneecap.

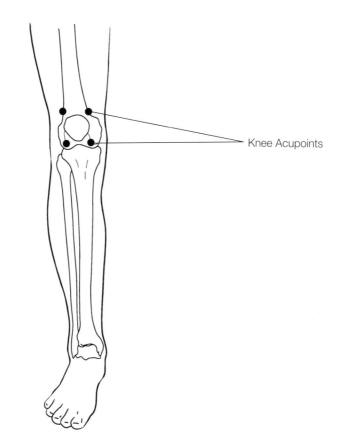

Knee Acupoints

Technique: Support the back of the knee with the fingers of both hands and locate the 2 points above the knee with the thumbs. Apply acupressure angled directly under the kneecap. Next, lower the thumbs to reach the 2 points below the kneecap and apply acupressure maintaining finger support behind the knees.

Benefits: Eases knee joint pain and relieves stiffness in the knees.

Urinary Bladder 40

Location: At the back of the knee, between the tendons.

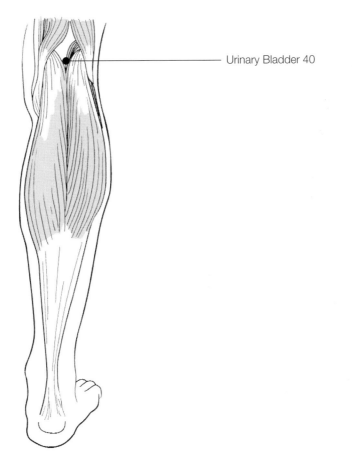

Urinary Bladder 40

Technique: Bend the knees slightly and place the thumbs at the side of the kneecaps for support and the fingers behind the knees. Locate the point with the index or middle fingers, feeling gently for the hollow in between the tendons. Do not press on the tendons themselves and avoid any varicose veins.

Benefits: Relieves pain in the knees and lower legs.

THE ANKLES

Maintain ankle mobility by regular ankle rotations and pointing and flexing the feet. Avoid standing for long periods and relieve swollen ankles by raising them for 15–20 minutes in the evening. Ankle pain may also be related to deficiency in the kidney and bladder meridians so relief may be obtained when these meridians are stimulated (see Urinary Health, pp. 177–88).

To relieve pain and stiffness in the ankles, add the following:

Kidney 3

Location: On the inside of the ankle in the depression level with the tip of the ankle bone.

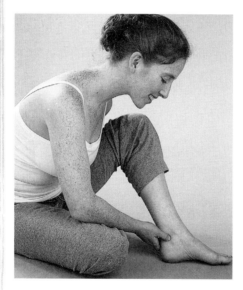

Technique: Place the fingers of the opposite hand behind the ankle for support and locate the point with the thumb. Apply pressure perpendicularly or use small rotations. Repeat on opposite foot.

Benefits: Strengthens the ankle and relieves ankle pain.

Gall Bladder 40

Location: On the outside of the ankle bone and the outer edge of the tendon.

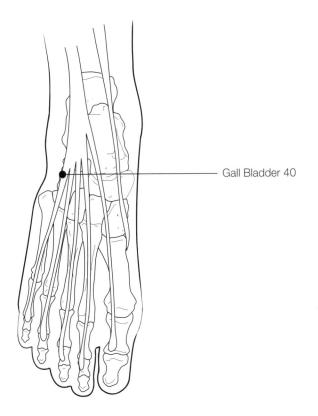

Gall Bladder 40

Technique: Place the fingers around the back of the ankle for support and locate the acupoint with the thumb. Apply acupressure angled slightly downwards towards the toes. Repeat on opposite foot.

Benefits: Reduces pain, swelling and weakness in the ankle joint.

If you have problems with your feet, you may find that massage and herbal foot baths will help. Avoid standing for long periods and elevate the legs for 10 minutes at the end of every day by placing the feet up against a wall or on a footstool with pillows. Comfortable shoes and moderate heels can also ease foot pain.

To relieve foot tiredness, pain or swelling, add the following:

Kidney 1

Location: A third of the way down the sole of the foot, in the depression just below the ball of the foot.

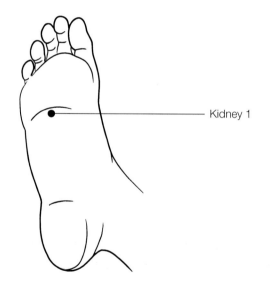

Kidney 1

Technique: Turn the sole of the foot upwards or sideways and support the foot with the fingers. Apply pressure perpendicularly, using one or both thumbs, one on top of the other. Repeat on other foot.

Benefits: Relieves aching feet and pain in the sole.

Gall Bladder 40

Location: On the outside of the ankle bone and the outer edge of the tendon.

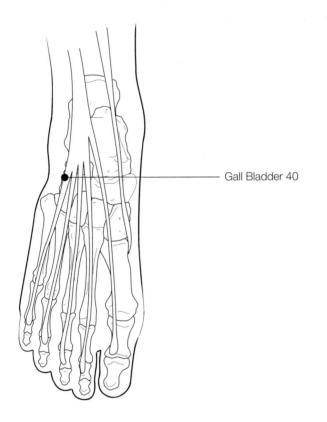

Gall Bladder 40

Technique: Place the fingers around the back of the ankle for support and locate the acupoint with the thumb. Apply acupressure angled slightly downwards towards the toes. Repeat on opposite foot.

Benefits: Relieves pain and swelling in the foot and ankle.

Urinary Bladder 60

Location: In the depression behind the ankle bone on the outside edge of the ankle.

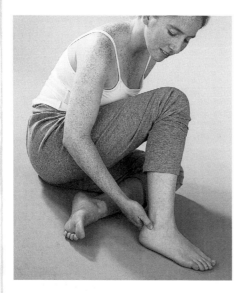

Technique: Place the right hand behind the right leg. Rest the fingers on the inside of the ankle for support and locate the acupoint on the outside edge of the ankle, using the thumb. Apply acupressure with the thumb angled slightly downwards towards the sole of the foot. Alternatively, if it is more comfortable, rest the thumb on the inside ankle and apply pressure with the index or middle finger. Repeat on opposite ankle.

Benefits: Relieves pain and swelling in the foot or heel.

Note: If pregnant, see pp. 10–11.

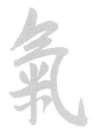

Healthy Lungs and Respiratory Function

Acupressure can be very effective in strengthening the lungs, improving breathing habits and in preventing and relieving common respiratory problems such as colds, bronchitis, coughing and asthma. It can also be helpful in stopping smoking.

The lungs can also be strengthened with regular breathing exercises. Yogic breathing exercises (*Pranayama*) are ideal (see Further Reading). At every opportunity, walk briskly in fresh air, breathing deeply. Regular aerobic exercise helps to improve lung function. Respiratory problems may be linked to food or inhalant allergies. Some people gain improvement by excluding dairy products from the diet, but professional allergy testing may be necessary to identify precise allergens. For chronic or severe respiratory problems you should consult your medical or complementary practitioner.

To strengthen the lungs and respiratory function, use the following acupoints on a regular basis:

Lung 7

Location: Two finger widths from the wrist crease closest to the palm on the inside of the forearm, in line with the thumb.

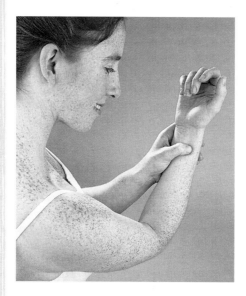

Technique: Support the wrist with the fingers of the opposite hand and locate the point with the thumb. Apply pressure angled down towards the thumb. Repeat on opposite wrist.

Benefits: Strengthens the lungs and respiratory system. Helps to prevent and relieve colds, coughs, congestion and breathing difficulties. This point may also be interchanged with Lung 9 (see p. 292).

Conception Vessel 17

Location: In the middle of the chest, in line with the nipples.

Technique: Locate the point with the middle or index finger of one hand and apply pressure perpendicularly against the breastbone, using gentle rotating movements.

Benefits: Stimulates lung function and relieves tension or pain in the chest.

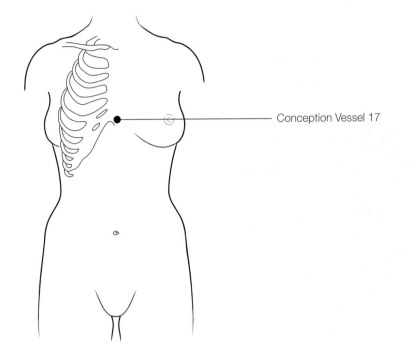

Conception Vessel 17

Respiratory Problems

THE COMMON COLD

At the first sign of a cold take rest, keep warm, drink plenty of fluids, avoid cold foods and dairy products and boost your vitamin C intake. The herb Echinacea boosts the immune system and helps prevent and ease colds. Add the following acupoints:

Governor Vessel 14

Location: At the back of the neck, between the seventh cervical vertebra and the first thoracic vertebra, approximately level with the shoulder.

Technique: Place one hand behind the neck and locate the point with the middle or index finger. Apply acupressure perpendicularly in the slight hollow between the vertebral joints.

Benefits: Prevents and relieves the common cold, fever, coughs, asthma and stiff necks.

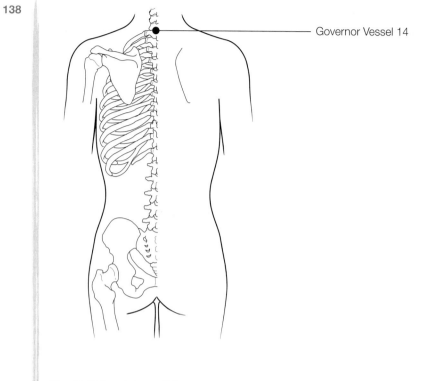

Governor Vessel 14

Gall Bladder 20

Location: At the back of the head, in the depression between the bottom of the skull and the neck muscles.

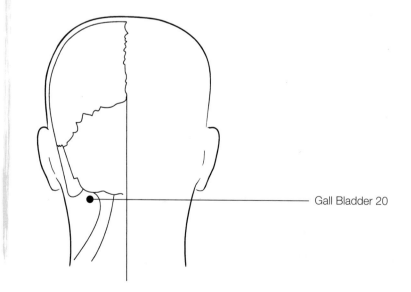

Gall Bladder 20

Technique: Rest the fingers on the back of the head and locate the point with the thumbs. Apply acupressure angled upwards under the edge of the skull on both sides of the spine.

Benefits: Prevents and relieves common colds, especially those caused by being out in the wind and cold.

Large Intestine 4

Location: In the centre of the triangle made by the bones of the thumb and the fingers. Can also be located at the end of the crease made by the index finger and thumb when they are pressed together.

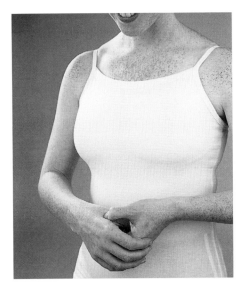

Technique: Support the palm of the left hand in the fingers of the right hand and locate the acupoint with the right thumb. Apply acupressure, angling the thumb slightly towards the wrist. Repeat on other hand.

Benefits: Can help to relieve some of the symptoms associated with common colds, such as nasal blockage and watery eyes.

Note: If pregnant, see pp. 10–11.

BRONCHITIS

To relieve the excess mucus, cough, wheeziness and breathlessness of bronchitis, add the following acupoints:

Conception Vessel 22

Location: In the depression below the throat, just above the top of the breastbone (sternum).

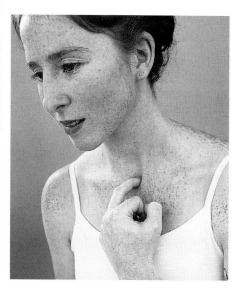

Technique: Locate the point with the middle or index finger of one hand and press in against the bone, not the windpipe.

Benefits: Helps to clear the throat and relieves coughs and hoarseness.

Location: Two finger widths on either side of the third thoracic vertebra, approximately level with the crest of the shoulder blade.

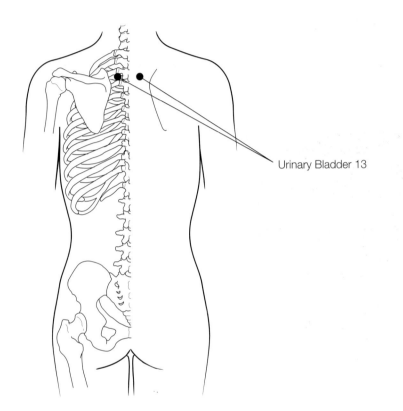

Urinary Bladder 13

Technique: Support the elbow in the opposite hand and reach over the shoulder to locate the point with the middle or index finger. Apply acupressure to the depression just below the wing of the vertebrae. Repeat on opposite side.

Benefits: Relieves coughing, fever and asthma. Helps to clear the lungs.

Add the following acupoint:

Lung 5

Location: On the inside of the elbow in the hollow on the outer edge of the tendons when the elbow is slightly bent.

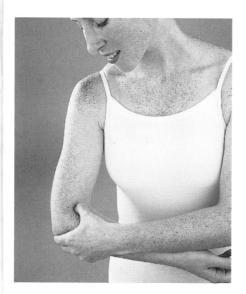

Technique: Support the elbow in the fingers of the opposite hand and locate the acupoint with the thumb. Apply acupressure perpendicularly and repeat on opposite arm.

Benefits: Relieves cough and constriction in the chest.

ASTHMA

Allergies often play a part in asthma and these should be professionally checked. Common allergens are dairy products, house dust and bed mites. Stress, anxiety, poor posture and bad breathing habits can also be significant factors. Some sufferers are helped by acupuncture and herbal medicine. Use of the special *Asthma Relief Acupoint* will help to prevent and abort asthma attacks, while *Stomach 40* helps reduce mucus and clear the airways.

Asthma Relief Acupoint

Location: At the back of the neck 1 finger width on either side of the spine at the junction between the seventh cervical vertebra and the first thoracic vertebra.

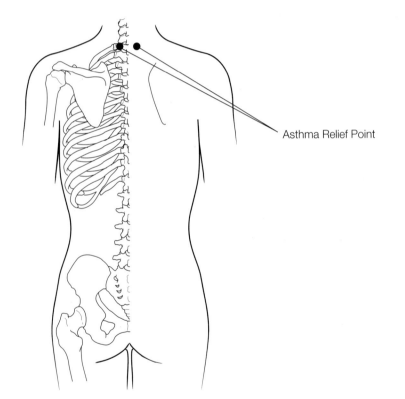

Asthma Relief Point

Technique: Place the hands over the shoulders and locate the point with the middle or index fingers. Apply acupressure firmly in the depression between the two vertebrae on either side of the spine.

Benefits: Frees the respiratory passages and relieves asthma.

Stomach 40

Location: On the outside edge of the leg bone halfway between the tip of the ankle bone and the middle of the kneecap.

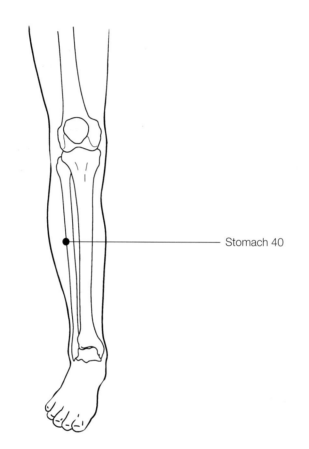

Stomach 40

Technique: Place the fingers behind the leg for support and apply acupressure using the thumbs.

Benefits: Helps to clear mucus in the respiratory passages and prevents and relieves asthma.

See also Nasal Problems (pp. 95–8), Chapter 13, Acupressure First Aid, Asthma Attack (pp. 287–9) and Asphyxia (pp. 291–3).

There are now many behavioural programmes, self-help books and videos available to help you give up smoking. It is important to identify the reasons why you smoke and the times of day and places you are most likely to smoke in order to change your habits.

An adequate supply of certain vitamins is also vital, especially vitamin C, B vitamins and chromium, which helps to balance the blood sugar levels that play an important part in cigarette craving.

The severe symptoms of nicotine withdrawal, cigarette craving and chest discomfort can all be reduced with acupressure, making giving up much easier as long as you have a sincere desire to quit. Use the following acupressure points as soon as you feel the need of a cigarette:

Ear Adrenal Acupoint

Location: On the border of the indentation (triangular fossa) of the upper ear.

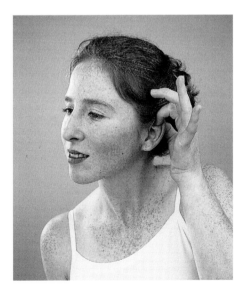

Technique: Stimulate the point gently with the smooth edge of a fingernail or a clean, pointed object such as a cocktail stick. Take care to apply only gentle pressure and not to damage the sensitive skin of the ear.

Benefits: Stimulates the adrenal system and helps to remove cigarette craving.

Lung 6

Location: On the forearm, just over halfway between the wrist and elbow in line with the thumb.

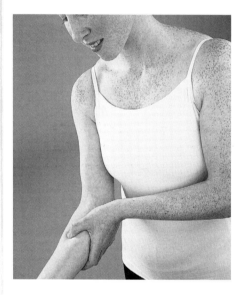

Technique: Support the lower arm with the fingers and locate the acupoint with the thumb. Apply acupressure angled slightly downwards towards the wrist. Repeat on opposite arm.

Benefits: Opens the chest and helps to detoxify and clear the lungs.

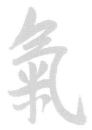

A Healthy Heart

A healthy heart and good circulation depend on regular exercise, good diet and effective stress management. Good circulation is crucial for maintaining comfortable body temperature, normal blood pressure, good complexion and hair and mobile joints. Dietary factors known to be important are the regulation of cholesterol levels, a reduced intake of saturated fats and salt and daily intake of essential fatty acids (EFA's) found in fish and plant oils. Increased fibre, whole grains, fresh fruit and vegetables and garlic are also helpful. People with heart or blood pressure problems should avoid smoking or drinking excessive alcohol or caffeine. Exercise should be moderate and regular, combined with relaxation and stress relief.

Acupressure can be very effective in strengthening heart function and promoting good circulation throughout the body. General points to tone the heart and stimulate circulation are as follows:

Heart 7

Location: On the outside edge of the wrist crease closest to the palm, in the hollow in line with the little finger.

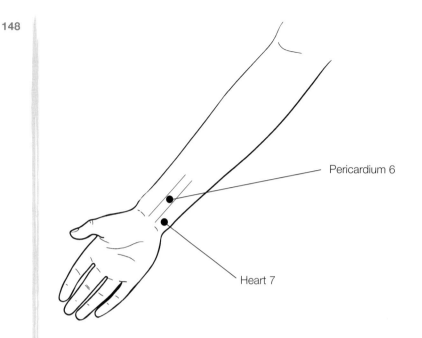

Pericardium 6

Heart 7

Technique: Turn the palm upwards and support the wrist in the fingers of the opposite hand. Locate the point with the thumb and apply pressure angled downwards towards the little finger. Repeat on opposite hand.

Benefits: Improves circulation, strengthens heart function and calms the mind.

Pericardium 6

Location: Between the tendons on the inside of the arm, 3 finger widths above the wrist crease closest to the palm.

Technique: Measure up from the wrist crease to locate the point. Support the wrist with the fingers of the opposite hand and apply acupressure to the point using the thumb, angled downwards towards the middle finger. Repeat on opposite hand.

Benefits: Strengthens the heart and improves circulation, especially in the arms and chest.

Stomach 36

Location: Four finger widths below the kneecap on the outside edge of the leg bone (tibia).

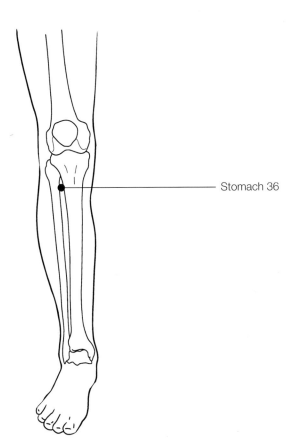

Stomach 36

Technique: Place the fingers behind the leg for support and locate the acupoint with the thumb. Apply acupressure angled slightly downwards towards the foot. Repeat on opposite leg.

Benefits: This is a general tonic point that improves circulation in the whole body.

acupressure

the heart and
circulation

Heart and Circulation Problems

Problems with the heart and circulation can be prevented or treated with acupressure as follows:

ANGINA AND PALPITATIONS

Use the heart acupoints already given on a daily basis and add the following points. Regular use of these points helps to improve the blood supply to the heart and prevent palpitations and angina. However, medical advice should always be sought for those with heart conditions.

Begin by using the points gently for short periods of time (just a few seconds each) and slowly build up to 5–10 seconds per point. Do not overstimulate the points and if you feel giddy or unwell stop immediately.

Conception Vessel 17

Location: In the middle of the chest, in line with the nipples.

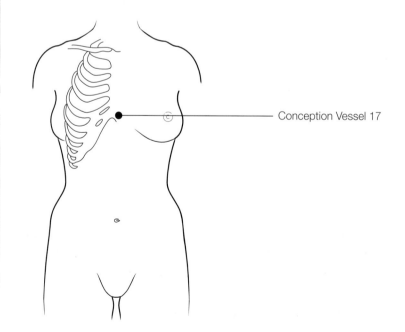

Conception Vessel 17

Technique: Locate the point with the middle or index finger and apply pressure perpendicularly against the breastbone, using gentle rotating movements.

Benefits: Increases circulation and relieves pain or palpitations in the chest.

Urinary Bladder 15

Location: Two finger widths on either side of the spine, level with the fifth thoracic vertebra (approximately halfway between the shoulder blades).

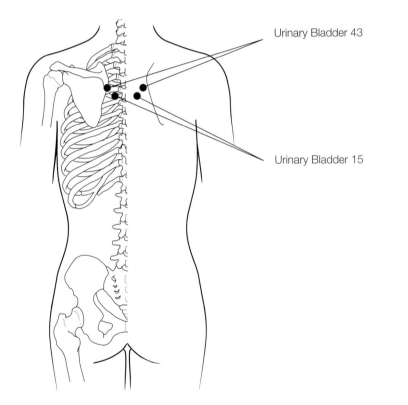

Urinary Bladder 43

Urinary Bladder 15

Technique: Reach over the opposite shoulder and apply acupressure with the index or middle finger. Repeat on other side. Alternatively lie on the ground and position two tennis balls level with the points and then press the back into them.

Benefits: Improves heart function and relieves palpitations and anxiety.

Urinary Bladder 43

Location: On the edge of the shoulder blade 4 finger widths on either side of the spine, level with the fourth thoracic vertebra.

Technique: As for *Urinary Bladder 15* (previous page).

Benefits: Releases tension in the chest and eases palpitations and anxiety.

Heart 3

Location: On the inside of the elbow at the end of the crease when the elbow is flexed.

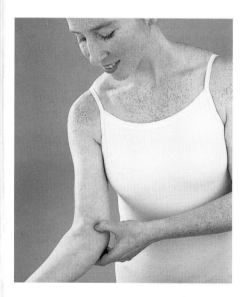

Technique: Support the elbow in the fingers of the opposite hand and locate the point using the thumb. Apply acupressure angled slightly downwards towards the little finger. Repeat on opposite arm.

Benefits: Relieves cardiac pain, numbness of the arm and constriction in the chest.

Pericardium 4

Location: On the inside of the forearm, just under halfway between the wrist and the elbow, in line with the middle finger, in the depression between the tendons.

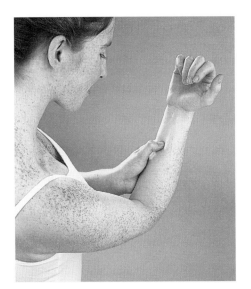

Technique: Rest the forearm in the fingers of the opposite hand and locate the point with the thumb. Apply acupressure angled slightly downwards towards the middle finger. Repeat on other hand.

Benefits: Relieves cardiac pain and palpitations by stimulating the blood supply to the coronary arteries.

POOR CIRCULATION IN THE HANDS AND FEET

To improve circulation, cut down on tea, coffee and smoking, which cause the blood vessels to constrict, and avoid sitting or standing for long periods. Regular gentle exercise, such as walking, and gentle rotations of the wrists and ankles may help. Daily vitamin C plus bioflavinoids and essential fatty acids (from fish or plant oils) are helpful, as is the herb Ginko biloba. Keep hands and feet warmly wrapped in cold weather and don't walk barefoot on cold floors or handle very cold implements such as ice trays. Use the general heart points and add the following:

acupressure

the heart and

circulation

Large Intestine 10

Location: On the forearm approximately 3 finger widths below the crease of the elbow in line with the point *Large Intestine 11* (see pp. 122) and the thumb.

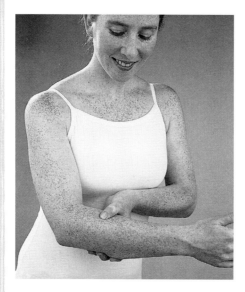

Technique: Support the elbow in the fingers of the opposite hand and locate the point using the thumb. Apply acupressure angled slightly downwards towards the thumb. Repeat on other arm.

Benefits: Improves circulation in the arm and upper body.

Gall Bladder 40

Location: On the outside of the ankle bone and the outer edge of the tendon.

Technique: Place the fingers around the back of the ankle for support and locate the acupoint with the thumb. Apply acupressure angled slightly downwards towards the toes. Repeat on opposite foot.

Benefits: Improves circulation in the feet and lower legs.

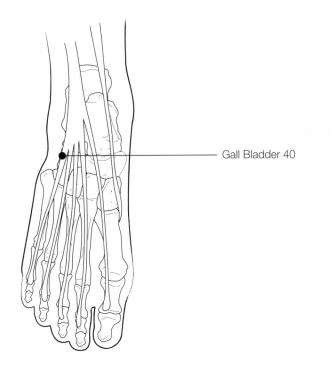

Gall Bladder 40

Kidney 3

Location: On the inside of the ankle in the depression level with the tip of the ankle bone.

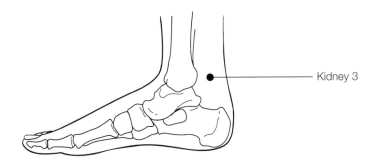

Kidney 3

Technique: Place the fingers of the opposite hand behind the ankle for support and locate the point with the thumb. Apply pressure perpendicularly or use small rotations. Repeat on opposite ankle.

Benefits: Improves circulation in the feet and lower body.

| Conception Vessel 4

Location: On the midline of the abdomen 4 finger widths below the navel.

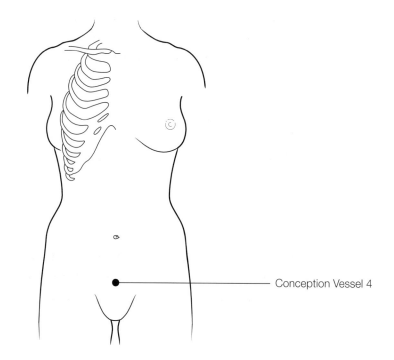

Conception Vessel 4

Technique: Measure 4 finger widths distance below the navel with one hand and locate the point with the middle or index finger of the opposite hand. Apply acupressure perpendicularly below the skin (apply only very light pressure if you are menstruating) and use gentle rotations to maintain the pressure.

Benefits: Improves circulation in the abdomen and lower body.

Note: If pregnant, see pp. 10–11.

High blood pressure may be prevented or reduced by stress management, relaxation and dietary changes. These include eliminating or decreasing intake of meat, alcohol, tea, coffee, saturated fats and refined sugars and increasing intake of essential fatty acids (EFAs), garlic, vitamin E and chromium. Chelation therapy has helped some sufferers. Low blood pressure, not generally recognized as a health problem, can cause fatigue and lethargy. Acupuncture and moxibustion can help boost and balance low blood pressure.

The same acupressure points are used to regulate high or low blood pressure, as they have a homoeostatic effect on the body, but the pressure may vary (see overleaf). Add the following 2 acupoints to the general heart points described already:

Governor Vessel 20

Location: At the top of the head on the midline between the tops of the 2 ears and in line with the top of the nose. Locate the point by placing the thumbs on the top of each ear and stretching the middle fingers out to meet at the top of the head.

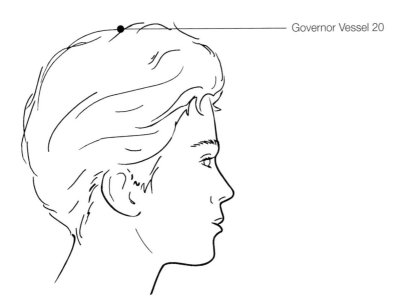

Governor Vessel 20

Technique: Apply acupressure perpendicularly into the scalp, using the middle or index fingertip. For firmer pressure you can rest the middle or index fingertip of the other hand on top of the nail of the finger locating the point and apply gentle pressure with both fingers simultaneously. The point should be felt as a small depression in the scalp and may feel slightly tender.

Benefits: Reduces dizziness and balances the blood pressure.

Caution: If you have high blood pressure do *not* overstimulate this point. Use only light pressure and stop immediately if you feel unwell or uncomfortable. For low blood pressure firm pressure may be used.

Kidney 1

Location: A third of the way down the sole of the foot, in the depression just below the ball of the foot.

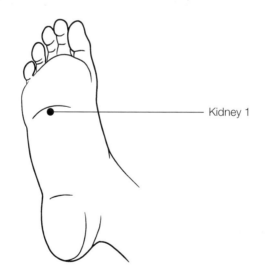

Kidney 1

Technique: Turn the sole of the foot upwards or sideways and support the foot with the fingers. Apply pressure perpendicularly, using one or both thumbs, one on top of the other. Repeat on opposite foot.

Benefits: Regulates blood pressure, relieves dizziness and faintness.

To relieve varicose veins, sit or lie down and raise your feet on pillows or against a wall several times during the day and especially before sleeping. Avoid constipation and try to lose weight if overweight. Support tights and low-heeled shoes may also help, as will showering the legs with alternating hot and cold water. Don't stand for long periods or cross the legs. Walk regularly. Applying witch hazel or calendula to the affected areas may also bring relief.

The following acupressure points will help improve flow of blood in the legs, but *never* apply acupressure on or near an actual varicose vein. If your leg is affected near to the acupressure point, use a point further along the same meridian line. Using the point on the opposite leg is still beneficial too.

Spleen 6

Location: On the inside of the leg, 4 finger widths above the tip of the ankle bone and just inside the bone of the leg (tibia).

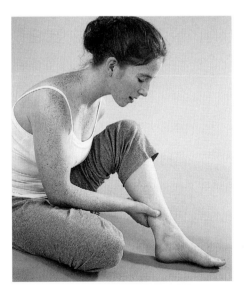

Technique: Measure up 4 fingers from the ankle bone with one hand and then use the thumb of the other hand to locate the acupoint. Apply acupressure perpendicularly and repeat on other leg.

Benefits: Improves circulation in the lower limbs.

Note: If pregnant, see pp. 10–11.

Spleen 10

Location: On the inside edge of the top of the knee, where the opposite thumb touches the muscle when the knee is flexed.

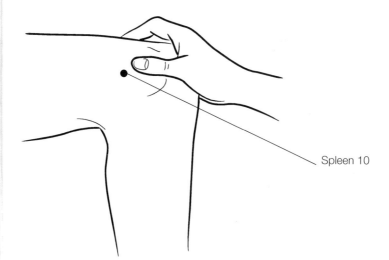

Spleen 10

Technique: Having located the acupoint with the opposite hand, replace it with the same hand, fingers resting on the outside of the knee and thumb applying pressure perpendicularly into the point. Repeat for other leg.

Benefits: Improves circulation in the legs.

See also Constipation, p. 165.

These may be prevented or relieved by improving posture, releasing neck and shoulder tension, improving general circulation and balancing blood sugar levels (low blood sugar can cause dizziness). Food allergy may also be a factor. The following additional points may be helpful:

Governor Vessel 20

Location: At the top of the head on the midline between the tops of the 2 ears and in line with the top of the nose. Locate the point by placing the thumbs on the top of each ear and stretching the middle fingers out to meet at the top of the head.

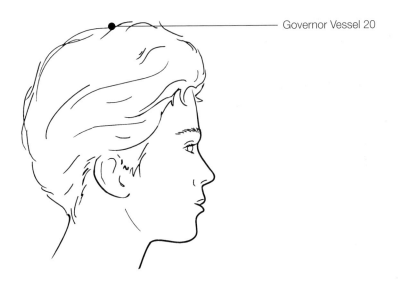

Governor Vessel 20

Technique: Apply acupressure perpendicularly into the scalp, using the middle or index fingertip. For firmer pressure you can rest the middle or index fingertip of the other hand on top of the nail of the finger locating the point and apply gentle pressure with both fingers simultaneously. The point should be felt as a small depression in the scalp and may feel slightly tender.

Benefits: Reduces dizziness and vertigo and balances blood pressure.

acupressure

the heart and

circulation

| # Kidney 3

Location: On the inside of the ankle in the depression level with the tip of the ankle bone.

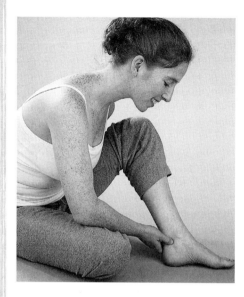

Technique: Place the fingers of the opposite hand behind the ankle for support and locate the point with the thumb. Apply pressure perpendicularly or use small rotations. Repeat on other foot.

Benefits: Strengthens the kidneys and relieves dizziness.

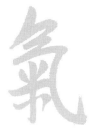

Healthy Digestion

Healthy digestion is a vital part of overall health. Acupressure can improve the functioning of the digestive organs and the absorption of food. The following points can be used regularly to maintain healthy digestion. However, do not use them right after eating or when very hungry. Gentle stimulation of the points before eating a meal will ensure good digestion afterwards.

Stomach 25

Location: On the abdomen 3 finger widths on either side of the navel.

Technique: Locate the point and apply acupressure using the index or middle fingers. Apply pressure perpendicularly into the abdomen on either side of the navel.

Benefits: Stimulates stomach and large intestine function and aids digestion.

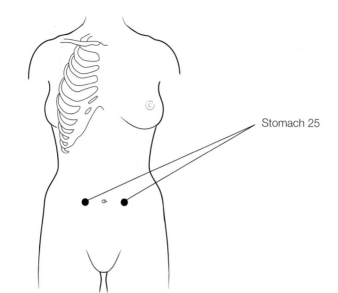

Stomach 25

Stomach 36

Location: Four finger widths below the kneecap on the outside edge of the leg bone (tibia).

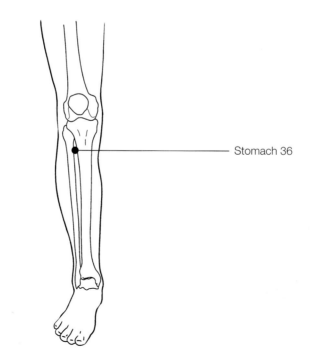

Stomach 36

Technique: Place fingers behind leg for support and locate acupoint with thumb. Apply acupressure angled slightly downwards towards foot. Repeat on opposite leg.

Benefits: Strengthens digestion and relieves indigestion and abdominal bloating.

Digestive Problems

Acupressure can prevent and relieve a wide range of digestive problems:

CONSTIPATION

Exercise regularly and drink plenty of water. Increase intake of fibre, found in wholemeal bread, brown rice and wholegrains, and of essential fatty acids (EFAs). Herbal remedies may also help.

Large Intestine 11

Location: In the depression at the end of the elbow crease, when the elbow is bent.

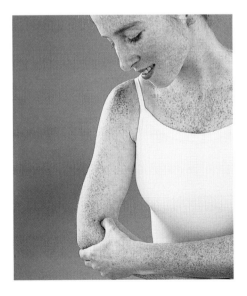

Technique: Support the elbow in the fingers and palm of the opposite hand and locate the point with the thumb. Apply acupressure angled slightly towards the elbow and upper arm. Repeat on other arm.

Benefits: Stimulates the large intestine and relieves constipation.

Large Intestine 4

Location: In the centre of the triangle made by the bones of the thumb and the fingers. Can also be located at the end of the crease made by the index finger and thumb when they are pressed together.

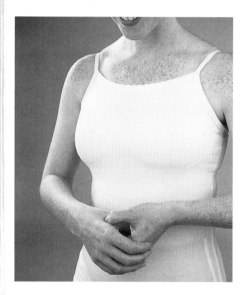

Technique: Support the palm of one hand in the fingers of the other and locate the acupoint with the thumb. Apply acupressure, angling the thumb slightly towards the wrist. Repeat for other hand.

Benefits: Relieves constipation and improves large intestine function.

Note: If pregnant, see pp. 10–11.

Location: Two finger widths on either side of the spine, level with the fourth lumbar vertebra and crest of the hipbones.

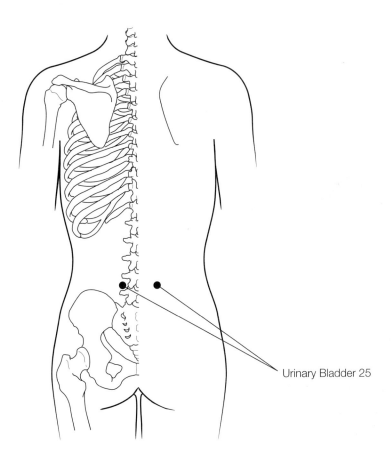

Urinary Bladder 25

Technique: Place the thumbs around the hips and locate the point with the middle fingers, applying acupressure deep into the tissue.

Alternatively, lie on the floor and apply pressure using the knuckles or tennis balls.

Benefits: Relieves constipation and abdominal pain or blockage.

acupressure

digestion

DIARRHOEA

This can be due to many causes, including anxiety, food allergy, food poisoning, repeated use of antibiotics or bowel disease. Drink plenty of water, as diarrhoea dehydrates the body. The following point can help but if symptoms persist seek medical advice.

Stomach 25

Location: On the abdomen 3 finger widths on either side of the navel.

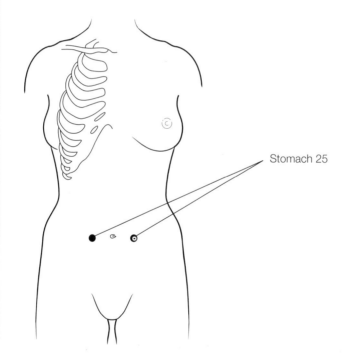

Stomach 25

Technique: Locate the point and apply acupressure using the index or middle fingers. Apply pressure perpendicularly into the abdomen on both sides of the navel.

Benefits: Balances digestion and relieves diarrhoea.

Stomach 34

Location: Three finger widths above the kneecap in the depression on the outer edge of the muscle.

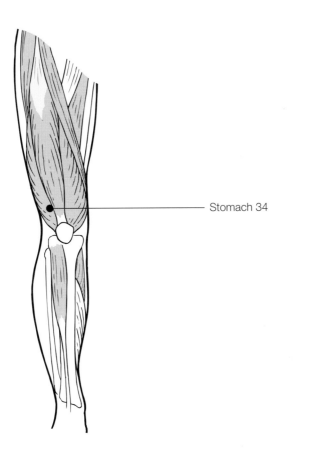

Stomach 34

Technique: Support knee with fingers and locate the acupoint with thumb. Apply acupressure angled slightly downwards towards knee. Repeat on other leg.

Benefits: Relieves digestive pain and discomfort and eases diarrhoea.

ABDOMINAL PAIN AND STOMACH CRAMPS

To relieve these conditions, study and modify your diet. Avoid acidic, sugary, yeasty and dairy foods and chew food slowly. Consider food intolerance testing. Relief of stress and anxiety is also important. If pain persists, seek medical advice. Add the following acupoints:

Stomach 34

Location: See previous page.

Technique: See previous page.

Benefits: Relieves abdominal pain and cramps.

Urinary Bladder 21

Location: Two finger widths on either side of the spine, level with the twelfth thoracic vertebra (approximately level with the lower end of the ribs).

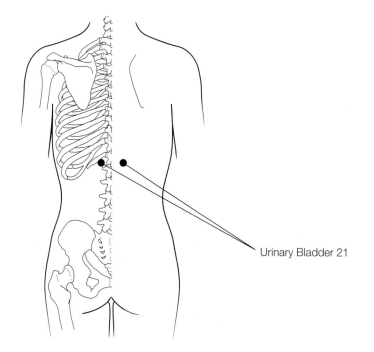

Urinary Bladder 21

Technique: Reach arms around to the back and apply acupressure using middle fingers, thumbs or knuckles. Or, lie on the floor and place the knuckles or two tennis balls in line with the acupoint and gradually lower spine onto them to apply pressure.

Benefits: Relieves abdominal swelling, indigestion and pain and stimulates the digestive organs, especially the stomach.

Spleen 8

Location: On the inside of the lower leg 4 finger widths below the knee in the depression underneath the bone.

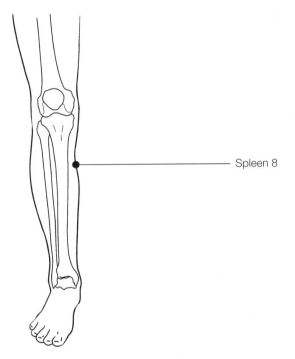

Spleen 8

Technique: Measure 4 finger widths down from the knee with the hand on the same side as the leg. Then using the opposite hand, place the fingers around the front of the leg and locate the acupoint with the thumb. Apply pressure angled slightly upwards towards the kneecap. Repeat on other leg.

Benefits: Balances digestion and relieves acute abdominal pain or swelling.

Appetite may be affected by psychological or emotional factors or nutritional factors such as zinc deficiency. To balance the appetite, whether you suffer from loss of appetite (anorexia) or over-eating, add the following acupoints:

Conception Vessel 12

Location: On the midline of the abdomen, halfway between the navel and the edge of the breast bone.

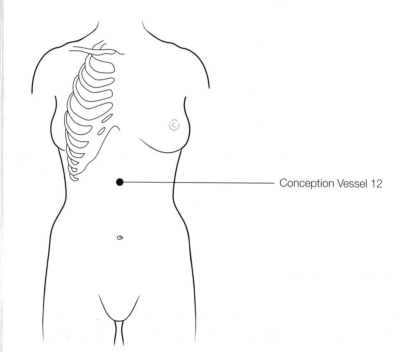

Conception Vessel 12

Technique: Apply acupressure perpendicularly, using either the index or middle finger.

Benefits: Balances digestion and regulates the appetite.

Location: On the border of the indentation (triangular fossa) of the upper ear.

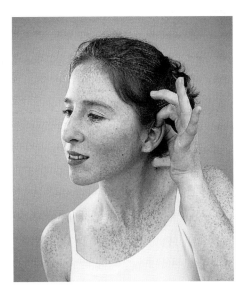

Technique: Stimulate the point gently with the smooth edge of a fingernail or a clean, pointed object such as a cocktail stick. Take care to apply only gentle pressure and not to damage the sensitive skin of the ear.

Benefits: Regulates the appetite.

NAUSEA AND TRAVEL SICKNESS

Ginger is effective in reducing nausea and travel sickness. Take as a lozenge or an infusion together with honey and grated lemon peel (from a non-waxed lemon). This beverage also reduces early-morning nausea.

The following acupoint is superior to any other for temporary nausea and travel sickness and should be stimulated continuously until the nausea subsides. Alternatively, commercial acupoint wristbands that apply continuous pressure to the point are very effective (see Useful Addresses).

Pericardium 6

Location: Between the tendons on the inside of the arm, 3 finger widths above the wrist crease closest to the palm.

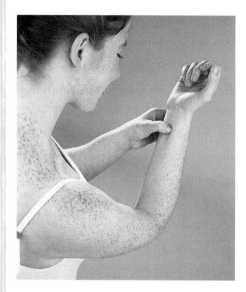

Technique: Measure up from the wrist crease to locate the point. Support the wrist with the fingers of the opposite hand and apply acupressure to the point using the thumb, angled downwards towards the middle finger. Repeat for opposite arm.

Benefits: Relieves nausea and travel sickness.

See also Travel Sickness (pp. 311–12).

To relieve flatulence, try cutting out dairy foods, bread, yeast and sugar. Food combinations may also be at fault (see Further Reading). The following acupoint can help:

Spleen 4

Location: On the inside of the foot in the depression behind the bone of the big toe.

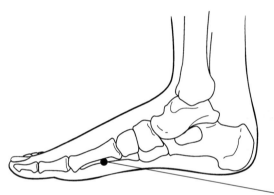

Spleen 4

Technique: Rest the fingers over the top of the foot and locate the acupoint with the thumb. Apply acupressure perpendicularly into the foot. Repeat on other foot.

Benefits: Balances the digestive organs; relieves abdominal bloating and flatulence.

HEARTBURN

Heartburn can be caused by too rapid eating, poor food combining, alcohol, tension and anxiety and being overweight. Avoid tight-fitting clothes, eat small meals slowly and chew well. Never accompany meals with alcohol, coffee or smoking. Don't lie down after meals and take regular exercise to improve digestive function.

Add the following acupoint:

Conception Vessel 12

Location: On the midline of the abdomen, halfway between the navel and the edge of the breast bone.

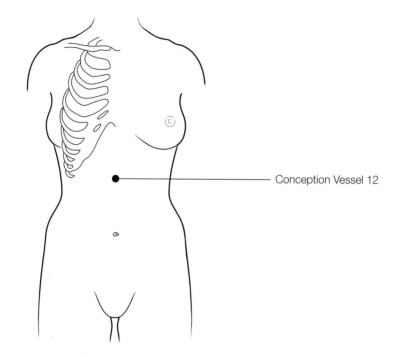

Conception Vessel 12

Technique: Apply acupressure perpendicularly, using either the index or middle finger.

Benefits: Relieves gastric pain.

FOOD POISONING

See Chapter 13, Acupressure First Aid, Food Poisoning (pp. 301–2).

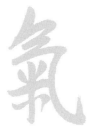

Urinary Health

In Oriental medicine the kidneys are seen as the source of both vitality and longevity, so great care is taken to strengthen and nourish them. In addition, as the kidneys and urinary bladder are important organs for detoxification and elimination, their healthy function is considered vital. To improve kidney function, drink plenty of good quality water every day and reduce coffee, tea, alcohol and sweet or spicy foods. Leafy greens, pulses and root vegetables all benefit the kidneys. Smoking does not; cut down or stop. Acupressure is widely used to improve and maintain kidney and bladder function and is very effective when used on a regular basis.

Urinary Bladder 23

Location: On the lower back 2 finger widths on either side of the spine, approximately level with the waist, by the lower edge of the second lumbar vertebra.

Technique: Place the thumbs on either side of the waist and locate the point on both sides of the spine using the middle fingers. Alternatively, lie on the floor and, arching the back slightly, place the knuckles or two tennis balls level with the points and then gently lower the back onto them.

Urinary Bladder 23

Urinary Bladder 28

Benefits: Improves kidney function.

Urinary Bladder 28

Location: In the lower back, 2 finger widths on either side of the sacrum, level with the second sacral holes.

Technique: Place the thumbs around the hips and locate the point using the index or middle fingers. Apply acupressure with the fingers or use the knuckles for stronger pressure. Alternatively, apply pressure by lying down onto the knuckles.

Benefits: Improves urinary bladder function and urinary control.

Kidney 3

Location: On the inside of the ankle in the depression level with the tip of the ankle bone.

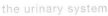

Technique: Place the fingers of the opposite hand behind the ankle for support and locate the point with the thumb. Apply pressure perpendicularly or use small rotations. Repeat on opposite foot.

Benefits: Improves kidney function, decreases frequent urination and relieves pain in the lower back related to weakness in kidney function.

Conception Vessel 3

Location: On the midline of the lower abdomen, about 1 hand width below the navel and 1 thumb width above the top of the pubic bone.

Technique: Locate the pubic bone, using the middle finger, and then, with the index finger, locate the acupoint just above. Apply acupressure perpendicularly.

Benefits: Improves bladder function, prevents urine retention and relieves frequent urination.

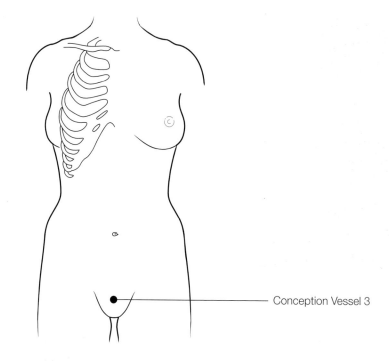

Conception Vessel 3

Urinary Problems

Weak kidney and bladder function can lead to urinary problems and water retention. It can also contribute to low back pain (see pp. 120–26), knee joint problems (see pp. 127–9), ear problems (see pp. 89–93), sore throats (see pp. 105–8) and certain gynaecological or sexual problems (see Chapters 8 and 9).

INVOLUNTARY URINATION (INCONTINENCE/BED-WETTING)

This may be caused by stress and anxiety or weak muscles. In women the pelvic floor muscles can be strengthened with simple pelvic floor exercises. For involuntary urination or too frequent urination, add:

Spleen 6

Location: On the inside of the leg, 4 finger widths above the tip of the ankle bone and just inside the bone of the leg (tibia).

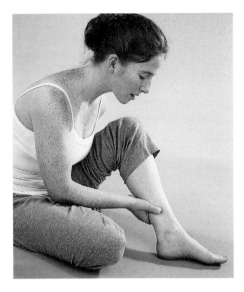

Technique: Measure up 4 finger widths from the ankle bone with one hand and then use the thumb of the other hand to locate the acupoint. Apply acupressure perpendicularly, and repeat on opposite leg.

Benefits: Regulates the functions of the bladder and kidneys and improves urinary control.

Note: If pregnant, see pp. 10–11.

Liver 1

Location: On the inside of the big toe at the corner of the toenail.

Technique: Stimulate using the edge of the nail of the thumb or index finger.

Benefits: Improves circulation in the lower abdomen and regulates bladder function.

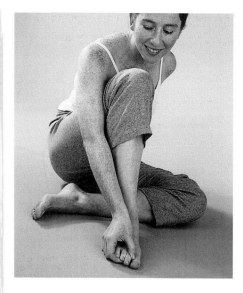

URINARY RETENTION

To relieve urinary retention and to prevent prostate trouble in men, add the following points. Acupuncture and herbal medicine can also be helpful. Zinc supplements, or plenty of zinc-rich foods such as pumpkin seeds and oysters, help prevent prostate trouble as does the herb Saw Palmetto. Coffee, tea, alcohol and cigarettes should be reduced, as they inhibit zinc absorption. Established prostate problems require medical attention.

Spleen 6

Location: On the inside of the leg, 4 finger widths above the tip of the ankle bone and just inside the bone of the leg (tibia).

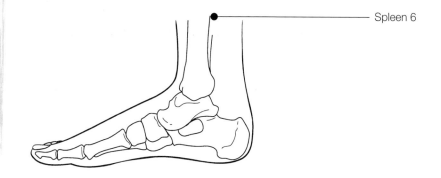

Spleen 6

Technique: Measure up 4 finger widths from the ankle bone with one hand and then use the thumb of the other hand to locate the acupoint. Apply acupressure perpendicularly and repeat on other leg.

Benefits: Regulates the function of the bladder and kidneys and improves urinary control.

Note: If pregnant, see pp. 10–11.

Gall Bladder 39

Location: On the outside of the leg 4 finger widths above the tip of the ankle bone in the depression between the bone and the tendons.

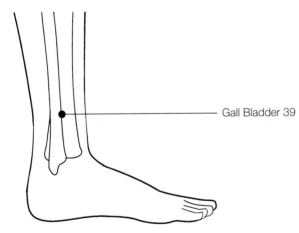

Gall Bladder 39

Technique: Place the fingers behind the leg for support and locate the point with the thumb. Apply acupressure angled slightly downwards towards the heel. Repeat on other leg.

Benefits: Improves circulation and the elimination of excess fluids from the body.

Stomach 28

Location: Four finger widths below the navel and 3 finger widths on either side of the midline of the abdomen.

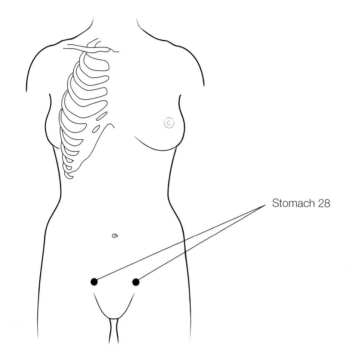

Stomach 28

Technique: Place the fingers on the sides of the abdomen and locate the point with the middle fingers. Apply acupressure angled slightly downwards towards the pelvis.

Benefits: Relieves abdominal blockage and promotes the release of urine.

WATER RETENTION AND SWELLING (OEDEMA)

To prevent oedema (water retention and swelling in the tissues), reduce salt intake as salt promotes the retention of fluids. Increase intake of natural diuretics which help to expel excess fluids from the body: parsley, celery and dandelion leaves are all excellent. Eat them raw or drink them as infusions in boiled water. Try the following acupoints:

Spleen 9

Location: Below the knee on the inside of the leg in the depression between the leg bone (tibia) and the muscle.

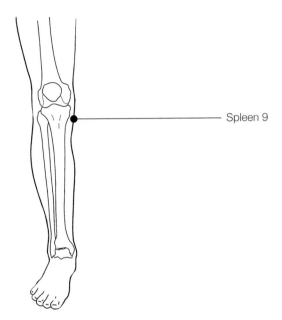

Spleen 9

Technique: Locate the acupoint with the thumb and apply acupressure perpendicularly. Repeat on other leg.

Benefits: Helps to expel excess fluid from the body.

Spleen 6

Location: On the inside of the leg, 4 finger widths above the tip of the ankle bone and just inside the bone of the leg (tibia).

Technique: Measure 4 finger widths up from the ankle bone with one hand and then use the thumb of the other hand to locate the acupoint. Apply acupressure perpendicularly and repeat on opposite leg.

Benefits: Improves circulation and expels excess fluids in the lower body.

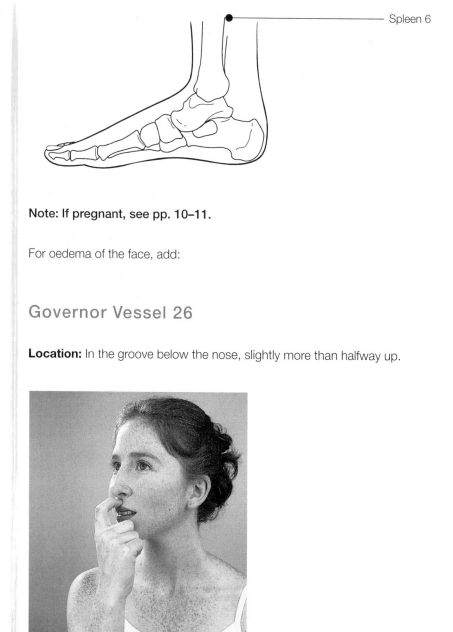

Spleen 6

Note: If pregnant, see pp. 10–11.

For oedema of the face, add:

Governor Vessel 26

Location: In the groove below the nose, slightly more than halfway up.

Technique: Locate the point with the nail edge or fingertip of the index or middle finger and place the thumb under the chin for support. Apply acupressure lightly, pressing perpendicularly against the gums underneath.

Caution: Do not overstimulate this point if you have high blood pressure; stop immediately if you feel unwell or uncomfortable.

Benefits: Relieves swelling of the face and helps expel excess fluid.

CYSTITIS/URINARY INFECTIONS

Cystitis can be prevented by a range of self-help measures (see Further Reading). These include drinking plenty of good quality water, avoiding excess coffee, tea and alcohol (especially spirits), keeping the lower body warm, wearing cotton underwear, wiping from front to back after urinating and always passing urine as soon as possible after sex. If you have needed antibiotics to treat acute cystitis, take a course of *Lactobacillus acidophilus* probiotics as soon as the course is complete to replace essential healthy bacteria. Acupressure, acupuncture, herbal medicine and homoeopathy are all helpful in preventing recurrent urinary infections. Add:

Stomach 28

Location: Four finger widths below the navel and 3 finger widths on either side of the midline of the abdomen.

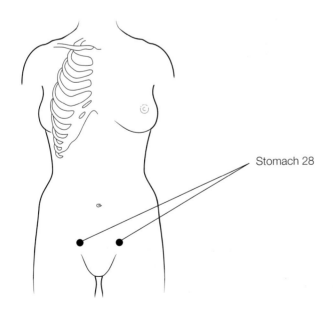

Stomach 28

Technique: Place the fingers on the sides of the abdomen and locate the point with the middle fingers. Apply acupressure angled slightly downwards towards the pelvis.

Benefits: Encourages urination and relieves abdominal discomfort.

Gall Bladder 25

Location: On the side of the abdomen level with the end of the twelfth rib.

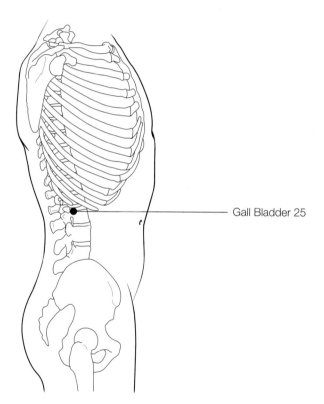

Gall Bladder 25

Technique: Place the thumb around the waist and locate the point with the index finger. Apply acupressure into the space under the rib. The point may be very tender, especially during a cystitis attack, so apply gentle, gradual pressure.

Benefits: Stimulates the kidneys and relieves urinary discomfort.

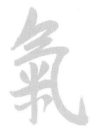

Gynaecological Health

Gynaecological health means trouble-free menstruation, pregnancy and menopause (see also Chapter 9, Sexual Health, pp. 209–18). In Oriental medicine gynaecological health is also thought to relate to vitality and longevity. Regular use of the following points will help to ensure healthy gynaecological function and build general vitality.

Additional acupressure points can be used to ease menstrual or menopausal discomfort and to facilitate pregnancy and birth (see Chapter 12, Pregnancy and Childbirth, pp. 265–84).

Conception Vessel 3

Location: On the midline of the lower abdomen, about 1 hand width below the navel and 1 thumb width above the top of the pubic bone.

Technique: Locate the pubic bone with the middle finger and then locate the acupoint just above with the index finger. Apply acupressure perpendicularly.

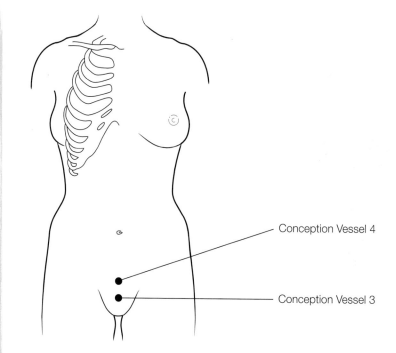

Conception Vessel 4

Conception Vessel 3

Benefits: Strengthens gynaecological function, regulates menstruation, clears discharge, prevents uterine prolapse.

Conception Vessel 4

Location: On the midline of the abdomen 4 finger widths below the navel.

Technique: Measure 4 finger widths below the navel with one hand and locate the point with the middle or index finger of the opposite hand. Apply acupressure perpendicularly below the skin (apply only very gentle pressure if menstruating).

Benefits: Improves gynaecological function, regulates menstruation and strengthens the uterus.

Note: If pregnant, see pp. 10–11.

Spleen 6

Location: On the inside of the leg, 4 finger widths above the tip of the ankle bone and just inside the bone of the leg (tibia).

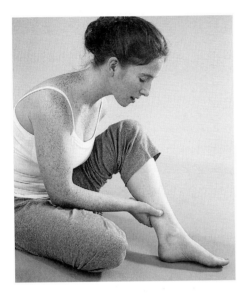

Technique: Measure 4 finger widths up from the ankle bone with one hand and then use the thumb of the other hand to locate the acupoint. Apply acupressure perpendicularly and repeat on opposite leg.

Benefits: Promotes fertility, regulates menstruation and relieves genital pain.

Note: If pregnant, see pp. 10–11.

Gynaecological Problems

MENSTRUAL IMBALANCE

If you suffer from menstrual problems, reduce sweet foods, dairy products, coffee, tea and alcohol in the week before your period, but keep your blood sugar level up by eating little and often. Boost your levels of vitamin C, iron, magnesium and zinc as all tend to fall before and during menses, paving the way for pain and fatigue.

acupressure

the gynaecologica

organs

Vitamin B6 and gamma linoleic acid found in Borage oil and Evening Primrose oil help ease menstrual pain. Stress and lack of exercise can contribute to menstrual imbalance.

PAINFUL OR HEAVY PERIODS

To prevent or ease painful or heavy periods (dysmenorrhoea), use the following points on a daily basis the week before your period is due:

Large Intestine 4

Location: In the centre of the triangle made by the bones of the thumb and the fingers. Can also be located at the end of the crease made by the index finger and thumb when they are pressed together.

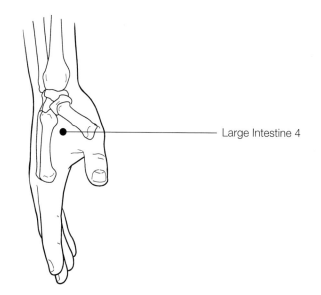

Large Intestine 4

Technique: Support the palm of the left hand in the fingers of the right hand and locate the acupoint with the right thumb. Apply acupressure, angling the thumb slightly towards the wrist. Repeat on other hand.

Benefits: Relieves blockage or pain in the lower abdomen.

Note: If pregnant, see pp. 10–11.

Spleen 8

Location: On the inside of the lower leg 4 finger widths below the knee in the depression underneath the bone.

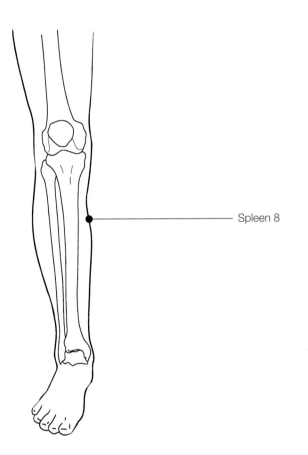

Spleen 8

Technique: Measure 4 finger widths down from the knee with the hand on the same side as the leg. Then, using the opposite hand, place the fingers around the front of the leg and locate the acupoint with the thumb. Apply pressure angled slightly upwards towards the kneecap. Repeat for other leg.

Benefits: Removes blockage in the lower abdomen and regulates menstruation.

acupressure

the gynaecological

organs

Spleen 10

Location: On the inside edge of the top of the knee, where the opposite thumb touches the muscle when the knee is flexed.

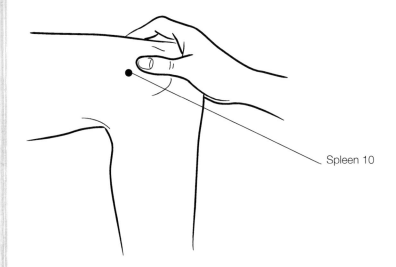

Spleen 10

Technique: Having located the acupoint with the opposite hand, replace it with the same hand, fingers resting on the outside of the knee and thumb applying pressure perpendicularly to the point. Repeat on the other leg.

Benefits: Improves blood circulation and relieves menstrual pain.

MENSTRUAL TIREDNESS AND BACK PAIN

To relieve menstrual tiredness and back pain, add:

Conception Vessel 6

Location: Two finger widths below the navel on the midline of the abdomen.

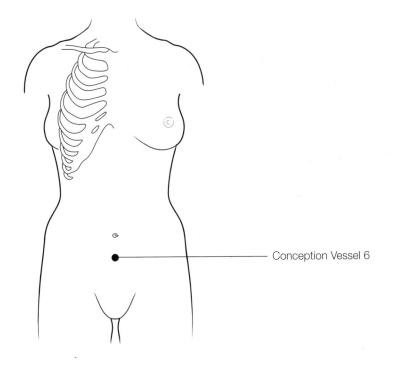

Conception Vessel 6

Technique: Place 2 fingers of one hand horizontally below the navel and locate the point using the middle or index finger of the other hand. Apply pressure perpendicularly and use gentle rotating movements with the fingertip.

Benefits: Promotes vitality and regulates menses.

Urinary Bladder 23

Location: On the lower back 2 finger widths on either side of the spine, approximately level with the waist, by the lower edge of the second lumbar vertebra.

Technique: Place the thumbs on either side of the waist and locate the point on both sides of the spine using the middle fingers. Alternatively, lie on the floor and, arching the back slightly, place the knuckles or two tennis balls level with the points and then gently lower the back onto them.

Benefits: Eases backache, regulates menses and stimulates the kidneys.

Urinary Bladder 23

Stomach 36

Location: Four finger widths below the kneecap on the outside edge of the leg bone (tibia).

Technique: Place the fingers behind the leg for support and locate the acupoint with the thumb. Apply acupressure angled slightly downwards towards the foot. Repeat for other leg.

Benefits: General tonic point that relieves tiredness and aching pains and builds vitality in the body.

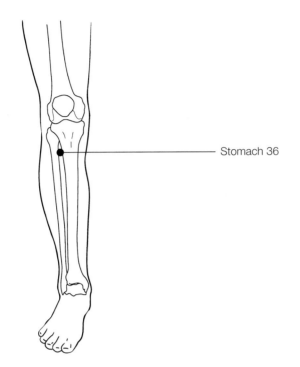

Stomach 36

ABSENCE OF PERIODS

For scanty or no menses (amenorrhoea), add:

Large Intestine 4

Location: In the centre of the triangle made by the bones of the thumb and the fingers. Can also be located at the end of the crease made by the index finger and thumb when they are pressed together.

Technique: Support the palm of the left hand in the fingers of the right hand and locate the acupoint with the right thumb. Apply acupressure, angling the thumb slightly towards the wrist. Repeat for other hand.

Benefits: A general tonic point that also promotes circulation of blood and vital energy (*chi*).

Note: If pregnant, see pp. 10–11.

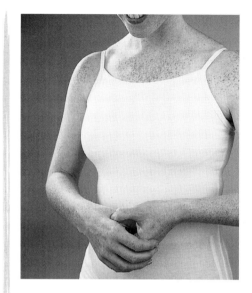

Spleen 10

Location: On the inside edge of the top of the knee, where the opposite thumb touches the muscle when the knee is flexed.

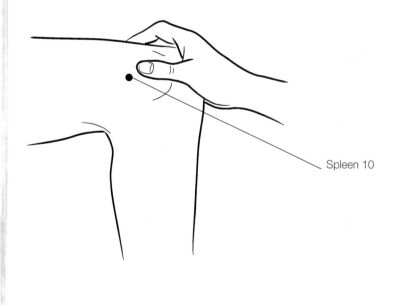

Spleen 10

Technique: Having located the acupoint with the opposite hand, replace it with the same hand, fingers resting on the outside of the knee and thumb applying pressure perpendicularly to the point. Repeat on the other leg.

Benefits: Promotes blood production and circulation.

Urinary Bladder 23

Location: On the lower back 2 finger widths on either side of the spine, approximately level with the waist, by the lower edge of the second lumbar vertebra.

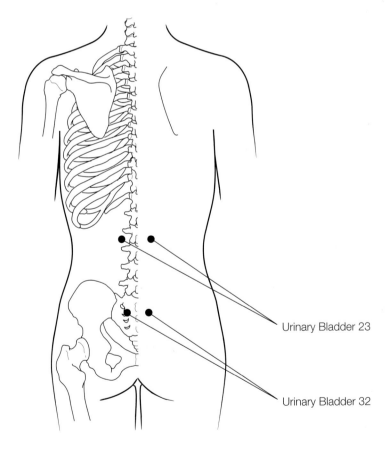

Urinary Bladder 23

Urinary Bladder 32

Technique: Place the thumbs on either side of the waist and locate the point on both sides of the spine using the middle fingers. Alternatively, lie on the floor and, arching the back slightly, place the knuckles or two tennis balls level with the points and then gently lower the back onto them.

Benefits: Improves kidney function and regulates menses.

Urinary Bladder 32

Location: At the base of the spine level with the second holes of the sacrum.

Technique: Place the thumbs across the base of the hips for support and locate the acupoint with the middle fingers. Apply pressure perpendicularly into the depression made by the sacral holes.

Benefits: Promotes blood flow in the uterus, regulates menses and relieves low back pain.

MENOPAUSAL IMBALANCE

A balanced diet, regular exercise, stress management, adequate rest and a positive attitude all help maintain health and vitality during the menopausal years. Good nutrition is vital. Mineral levels may become depleted during the menopausal years so a multi-mineral supplement can be helpful. Plant oestrogens, contained in soya products, can prevent or lessen hormonally related symptoms such as flushes and nightsweats. The herbs Agnus Castus, Black Cohosh and Mexican Yam are also useful. Ask a herbalist for specialist advice. Bone density can be maintained by regular weight-bearing exercise such as walking, jogging or skipping. Acupressure can help to ease some of the discomforts commonly associated with menopause.

HOT FLUSHES

For hot flushes, add:

Forehead Point (Extra Point)

Location: Above the bridge of the nose halfway between the inner edge of each eyebrow.

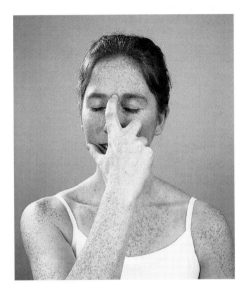

Technique: Locate with the index or middle fingertip of one hand, resting the thumb against the side of the face for support. Apply acupressure angled slightly downwards towards the bridge of the nose.

Benefits: Regulates hormonal changes and pituitary gland function; prevents and relieves hot flushes and headaches.

Large Intestine 4

Location: In the centre of the triangle made by the bones of the thumb and the fingers. Can also be located at the end of the crease made by the index finger and thumb when they are pressed together.

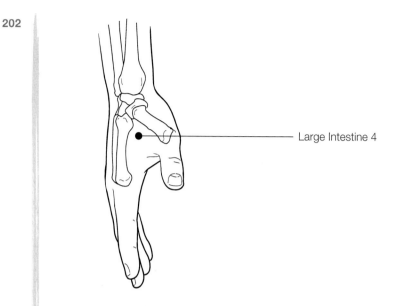

Large Intestine 4

Technique: Support the palm of the left hand in the fingers of the right hand and locate the acupoint with the right thumb. Apply acupressure, angling the thumb slightly towards the wrist. Repeat for other hand.

Benefits: Regulates blood circulation in the upper body and relieves heat in the head and face.

Note: If pregnant, see pp. 10–11.

Triple Heater 5

Location: On the outside of the forearm 3 finger widths above the wrist in the depression between the arm bones (radius and ulna).

Technique: Measure 3 finger widths from the wrist with the opposite hand. Locate the point with the index finger and support directly underneath the arm with the thumb. Apply acupressure perpendicularly. Repeat for other hand.

Benefits: Promotes circulation in the upper body and regulates body temperature. Can prevent and ease facial flushes.

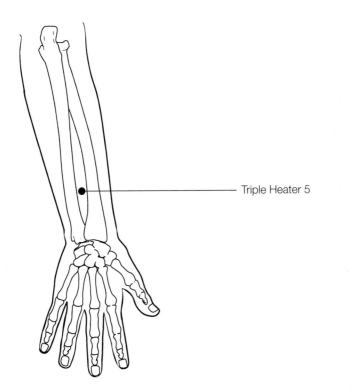

Triple Heater 5

Kidney 1

Location: A third of the way down the sole of the foot, in the depression just below the ball of the foot.

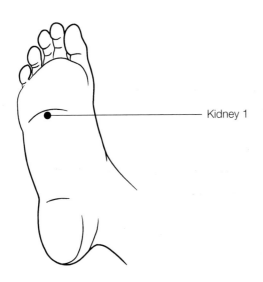

Kidney 1

Technique: Turn the sole of the foot upwards or sideways and support the foot with the fingers. Apply pressure perpendicularly, using one or both thumbs, one on top of the other. Repeat for other foot.

Benefits: Regulates blood pressure, clears the mind and relieves hot flushes.

MEMORY AND CONCENTRATION

To improve memory, concentration and emotional balance, add:

Governor Vessel 20

Location: At the top of the head on the midline between the tops of the 2 ears and in line with the top of the nose. Locate the point by placing the thumbs on the top of each ear and stretching the middle fingers out to meet at the top of the head.

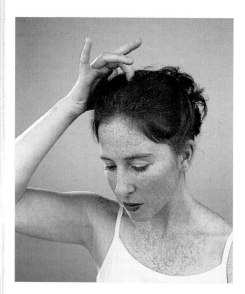

Technique: Apply acupressure perpendicularly into the scalp, using the middle or index fingertip. For firmer pressure you can rest the middle or index fingertip of the other hand on top of the nail of the finger locating the point and apply gentle pressure with both fingers simultaneously. The point should be felt as a small depression in the scalp and may feel slightly tender.

Benefits: Relieves congestion and blockage in the head and helps improve memory and concentration.

Note: Do not overstimulate this point if you suffer from high blood pressure.

Kidney 1

Location: A third of the way down the sole of the foot, in the depression just below the ball of the foot.

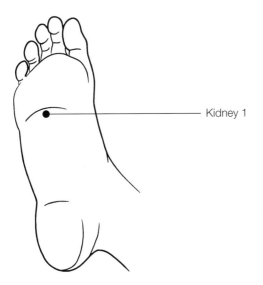

Kidney 1

Technique: Turn the sole of the foot upwards or sideways and support the foot with the fingers. Apply pressure perpendicularly, using one or both thumbs, one on top of the other. Repeat for other foot.

Benefits: Improves memory, concentration and mental alertness and helps relieve anxiety.

VAGINAL DRYNESS OR DISCHARGE

The same points treat both vaginal dryness or vaginal discharge because of their homoeostatic effect. Dryness may be helped by lubricants and ensuring plenty of essential fatty acids (such as fish and plant oils), oestrogen-rich soya products and vitamin E in the diet. Discharge should always be checked in case it is the result of infection or disease. However it is often due to candida or an after-effect of antibiotic treatment. This can be treated by avoiding all foods containing sugar, yeast, wheat and moulds and supplementing with probiotic healthy bacteria such as *Lactobacilus acidophilus*. Wearing cotton underwear and loose-fitting trousers or jeans will also help.

Conception Vessel 6

Location: Two finger widths below the navel on the midline of the abdomen.

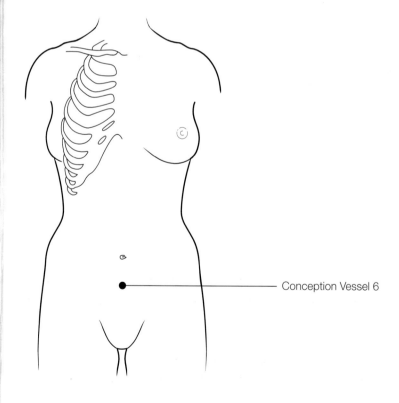

Conception Vessel 6

Technique: Place 2 fingers of one hand horizontally below the navel and locate the point using the middle or index finger of the other hand. Apply pressure perpendicularly and use gentle rotating movements with the fingertip.

Benefits: Improves gynaecological function and clears vaginal discharge.

Gall Bladder 26

Location: At the side of the abdomen, just below the eleventh rib and level with the navel.

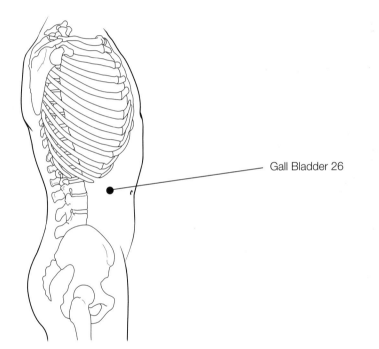

Gall Bladder 26

Technique: Place the fingers pointing downwards on the hips and locate the acupoint with the thumb. Apply acupressure angled into the abdomen and slightly downwards towards the pelvis.

Benefits: Regulates the flow of blood and *chi* (vital energy) in the lower abdomen. Reduces discharge and regulates menses. Regulates vaginal lubrication and can prevent dryness.

Governor Vessel 4

Location: On the spine, in the depression between the second and third lumbar vertebrae, approximately level with the waist.

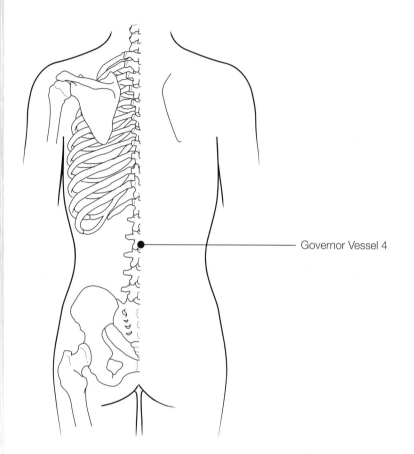

Governor Vessel 4

Technique: Place the thumb of one hand around the waist and use the middle finger to locate the point. Apply pressure gently in the space between the vertebrae.

Benefits: Regulates vaginal lubrication, prevents dryness and helps clear discharge. An important tonic point that strengthens gynaecological function.

See also Joint Problems (pp. 229–35), Poor Memory and Concentration (pp. 252–6), Urinary Health (pp. 177–88) and Sexual Health (pp. 209–18).

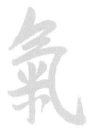

Sexual Health and Vitality

Sexual vitality is considered very important in Oriental medicine, not so much in terms of performance but rather in terms of the stimulation of the life-force in the body. Sexual energy used correctly is thought to charge all the organs of the body as well as to stimulate mental and spiritual functions. Weak sexual vitality or over-indulgence in sex can lead to a breakdown in health and both sexual and gynaecological problems. Mental, emotional and social factors, of course, also play an important role. Sexual energy, when strengthened, conserved and used wisely, is said to ensure longevity and good health.

Sexual health and vitality can be improved by regular exercise, adequate rest, stress management and adopting a healthy diet (increasing wholefoods, fresh fruit and vegetables and decreasing intake of nicotine, coffee and alcohol). Release of abdominal tension and increased circulation in the pelvic area are also important. These can be achieved by yoga exercises, postural work, massage and acupressure.

To build sexual vitality, the following acupressure points can be used 2 to 3 times a week and also before and after sexual contact if wished.

Conception Vessel 4

Location: On the midline of the abdomen 4 finger widths below the navel.

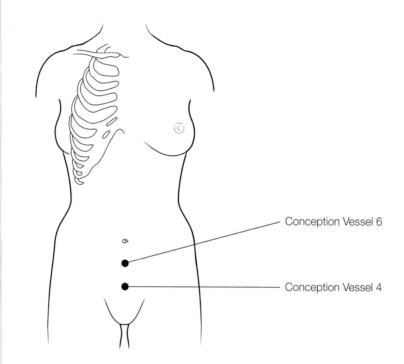

Conception Vessel 6

Conception Vessel 4

Technique: Measure 4 finger widths distance below the navel with one hand and locate the point with the middle or index finger of the opposite hand. Apply acupressure perpendicularly below the skin (apply only very gentle pressure if you are menstruating).

Benefits: Increases sexual potency and vitality, and strengthens gynaecological function.

Note: If pregnant see pp. 10–11.

Conception Vessel 6

Location: Two finger widths below the navel on the midline of the abdomen.

Technique: Place 2 fingers of one hand horizontally below the navel and locate the point using the middle or index finger of the other hand. Apply pressure perpendicularly and use gentle rotating movements with the fingertip.

Benefits: Increases energy levels and general vitality. Strengthens gynaecological function.

Note: If pregnant see pp. 10–11.

Governor Vessel 4

Location: On the spine, in the depression between the second and third lumbar vertebrae, approximately level with the waist.

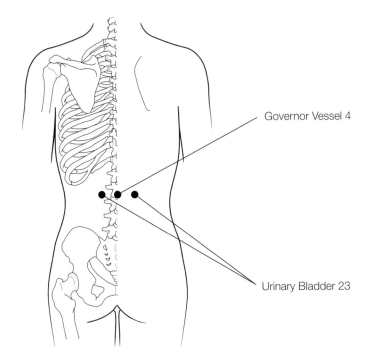

Governor Vessel 4

Urinary Bladder 23

Technique: Place the thumb around the waist and use the middle finger to locate the point. Apply pressure gently in the space between the vertebrae.

Benefits: Increases the strength of the kidneys, which are traditionally related to sexual vitality.

Urinary Bladder 23

Location: On the lower back 2 finger widths on either side of the spine, approximately level with the waist, by the lower edge of the second lumbar vertebra.

Technique: Place the thumbs on either side of the waist and locate the point on both sides of the spine using the middle fingers. Alternatively, lie on the floor and, arching the back slightly, place the knuckles or two tennis balls level with the points and then gently lower the back onto them.

Benefits: Strengthens the kidneys and improves sexual vitality.

Stomach 36

Location: Four finger widths below the kneecap on the outside edge of the leg bone (tibia).

Technique: Place the fingers behind the leg for support and locate the acupoint with the thumb. Apply acupressure angled slightly downwards towards the foot. Repeat for other leg.

Benefits: A general tonic point for increasing vitality in the body; strengthens the gynaecological and digestive organs.

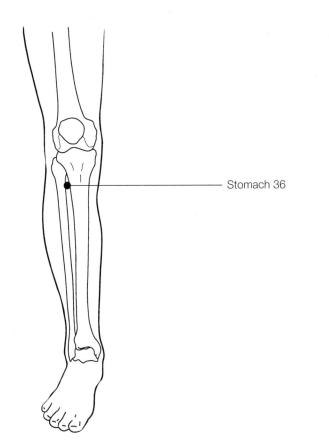

Stomach 36

Sexual Problems

Acupressure can help prevent and relieve sexual problems related to fatigue, low
sexual vitality or poor functioning of the sexual organs. However, mental, emotional,
dietary and environmental factors should always also be considered.

IMPOTENCE

Inability to obtain an erection is often accompanied by low back pain, general
listlessness, fatigue and anxiety. Using the sexual health acupoints on a daily basis
can help. The following acupoints may be added:

Governor Vessel 20

Location: At the top of the head on the midline between the tops of the 2 ears and in line with the top of the nose. Locate the point by placing the thumbs on the top of each ear and stretching the middle fingers out to meet at the top of the head.

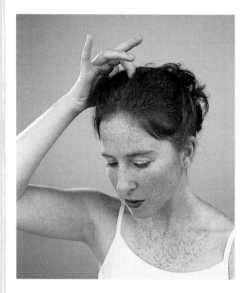

Technique: Apply acupressure perpendicularly into the scalp, using the middle or index fingertip. For firmer pressure, rest the middle or index fingertip of the other hand on top of the nail of the finger locating the point and apply gentle pressure with both fingers simultaneously. The point should be felt as a small depression in the scalp and may feel slightly tender. **Do not overstimulate if you have high blood pressure.**

Benefits: Raises energy in the body and can increase sexual vitality.

Kidney 3

Location: On the inside of the ankle in the depression level with the tip of the ankle bone.

Technique: Place fingers of the opposite hand behind the ankle for support and locate point with the thumb. Apply pressure perpendicularly or use small rotations. Repeat on other ankle.

Benefits: Strengthens the kidneys and the genitals.

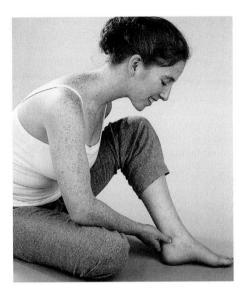

Heart 7

Location: On the outside edge of the wrist crease closest to the palm, in the hollow in line with the little finger.

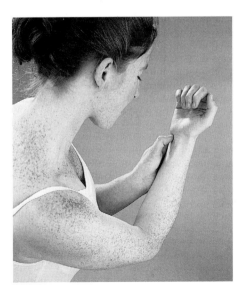

Technique: Turn the palm upwards and support the wrist in the fingers of the opposite hand. Locate the point with the thumb and apply pressure angled downwards towards the little finger.

Benefits: If the impotence is accompanied by anxiety, restlessness and insomnia, this point can be added to calm the mind and relieve anxiety.

SEMINAL EMISSION AND PREMATURE EJACULATION

Add the following points:

Kidney 3

Location: See page 214.

Technique: See page 214.

Benefits: Strengthens the kidneys and gynaecological function.

Urinary Bladder 52

Location: On the lower back 4 finger widths on either side of the spine level with the second lumbar vertebra (approximately level with the waist).

Technique: Place the thumbs around the waist and locate the acupoint with the middle fingers on either side of the spine. Apply pressure perpendicularly.

Benefits: Prevents seminal emission, increases sexual potency and relieves stiffness or pain in the lower back.

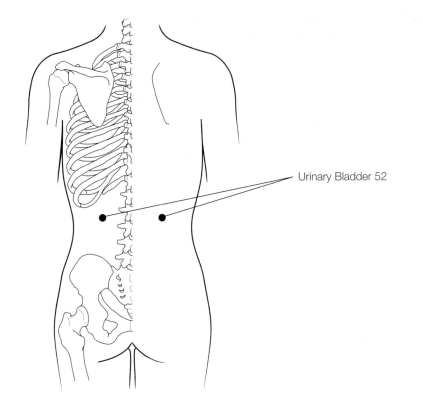

Urinary Bladder 52

SEXUAL APATHY AND PAIN

A lack of interest in sex and tension, anxiety, discomfort or even pain during intercourse, in either women or men, are closely connected with emotional issues and the relationship between sexual partners. However, these conditions can also be affected by weak sexual energy. This can be improved by daily use of the sexual health acupoints with the addition of the following points:

Kidney 3

Location: See page 214.

Technique: See page 214.

Benefits: Improves sexual vitality and relieves anxiety.

Spleen 6

Location: On the inside of the leg, 4 finger widths above the tip of the ankle bone and just inside the bone of the leg (tibia).

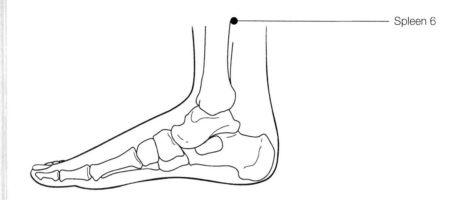

Spleen 6

Technique: Measure 4 finger widths up from the ankle bone with one hand and then use the thumb of the other hand to locate the acupoint. Apply acupressure perpendicularly. Repeat on opposite leg.

Benefits: Relieves genital and abdominal pain and strengthens gynaecological function.

Note: If pregnant, see pp. 10–11.

See also Chapter 7, The Urinary System, pp. 177–88 and Chapter 8, The Gynaecological Organs, pp. 189–208.

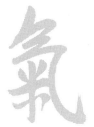

In the Acupressure Workout (pp.15–37) acupressure points were given for improving the function of each specific internal organ and body system. Additional points can be useful when an imbalance affects the body more generally, such as skin problems, aching muscles, joint problems, allergies or low immunity.

SKIN PROBLEMS

If you have problems with your skin, check that skin creams, medicated products, strong soap powders, environmental irritants or specific foods are not triggering your attacks. You can do this by keeping a careful diary of when skin problems occur, are at their worst and are improved. Food intolerance testing may also be useful (see Useful Addresses section). Common triggers are dairy products, shellfish and certain food additives. An imbalanced diet high in fatty or junk foods may also be a factor. Homoeopathic remedies are often helpful and noted success in eliminating skin problems has been achieved with Chinese herbs (see Useful Addresses section).

Skin irritation (hives), eczema and psoriasis can be relieved using the following points:

Large Intestine 4

Location: In the centre of the triangle made by the bones of the thumb and the fingers. Can also be located at the end of the crease made by the index finger and thumb when they are pressed together.

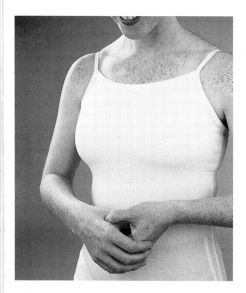

Technique: Support the palm of the left hand in the fingers of the right hand and locate the acupoint with the right thumb. Apply acupressure, angling the thumb slightly towards the wrist. Repeat on other hand.

Benefits: Relieves itching and helps to purify the blood.

Note: If pregnant, see pp. 10–11.

Conception Vessel 12

Location: On the midline of the abdomen, halfway between the navel and the edge of the breast bone.

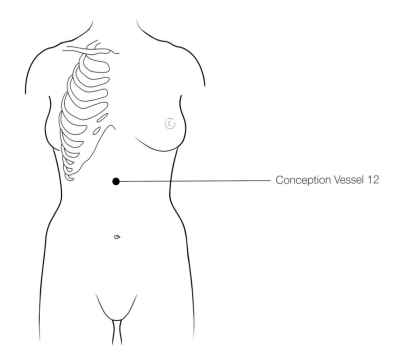

Conception Vessel 12

Technique: Apply acupressure perpendicularly, using either the index or middle finger.

Benefits: Can relieve digestive sensitivity and skin reactions due to food allergies.

Urinary Bladder 18

Location: 2 finger widths on either side of the spine, level with the ninth thoracic vertebra.

Technique: Lie on the floor with the knees bent and place either the knuckles or two tennis balls under the back, level with the point. Gradually lower the weight of the back onto the knuckles or balls to apply pressure to the point.

Benefits: Strengthens the liver and helps to purify the blood and detoxify the body, leading to improvement in skin conditions.

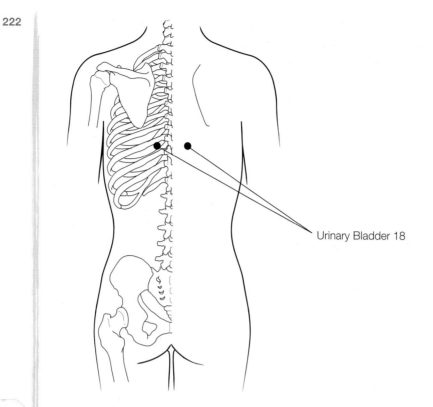

Urinary Bladder 18

Spleen 10

Location: On the inside edge of the top of the knee, where the opposite thumb touches the muscle when the knee is flexed.

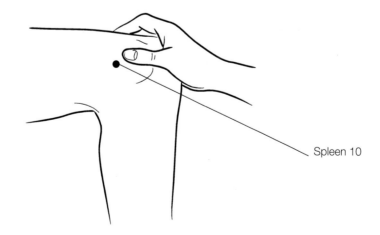

Spleen 10

Technique: Having located the acupoint with the opposite hand, replace it with the same hand, fingers resting on the outside of the knee and thumb applying pressure perpendicularly to the point. Repeat on the other leg.

Benefits: Regulates the blood and circulation and relieves skin irritation.

MUSCULAR PROBLEMS

Aching muscles and cramps can be relieved by gently extending the affected area and applying acupressure, massage and gentle stretching. For example, cramp in the calf muscles of the lower leg can be relieved by stretching the heel downwards and the toes upwards. If the cramp is due to water or salt loss (for example through excess sweating with exercise), then drink plenty of fluids including drinking water with a sprinkling of salt. However *never* give salt water to babies or young children as their kidneys are not fully developed and this can be fatal. If due to chilling, wrap and warm the body thoroughly. The homoeopathic remedy Mag. Phos. can also help prevent and relieve cramps.

To relieve cramps in the legs, add the following:

Urinary Bladder 40

Location: At the back of the knee, between the tendons.

Technique: Bend the knees slightly and place the thumbs at the side of the kneecaps for support and the fingers behind the knees. Locate the point with the index or middle fingers, feeling gently for the hollow in between the tendons. Do not press on the tendons themselves and avoid any varicose veins.

Benefits: Relieves cramps, tension and pain in the legs.

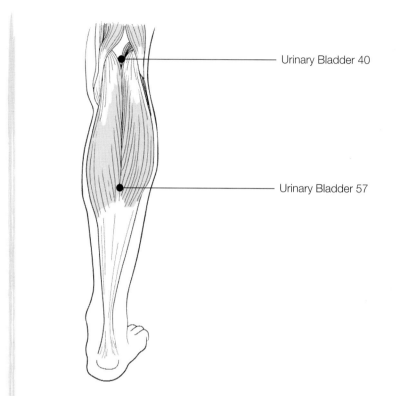

Urinary Bladder 40

Urinary Bladder 57

Urinary Bladder 57

Location: In the depression underneath the large muscle at the back of the leg (gastrocnemius).

Technique: Place the thumb on the side of the leg for support and locate the point with the middle or index finger. Apply acupressure angled slightly downwards towards the heel. Repeat for other leg.

Benefits: Releases spasm or pain in the muscles of the lower legs.

Spleen 9

Location: Below the knee on the inside of the leg in the depression between the leg bone (tibia) and the muscle.

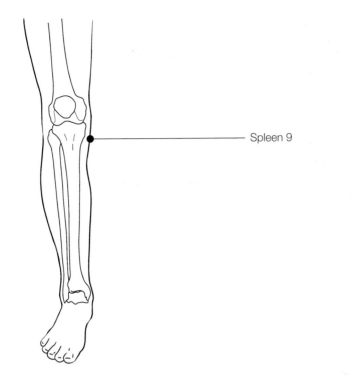

Spleen 9

Technique: Locate the acupoint with the thumb and apply acupressure angled slightly upwards towards the kneecap. Repeat on other leg.

Benefits: Relieves pain or spasm around the knees and lower legs.

For cramp in the hands, use the following acupoint:

Large Intestine 4

Location: In the centre of the triangle made by the bones of the thumb and the fingers. Can also be located at the end of the crease made by the index finger and thumb when they are pressed together.

Technique: Support the palm of the left hand in the fingers of the right hand and locate the acupoint with the right thumb. Apply acupressure, angling the thumb slightly towards the wrist. Repeat on opposite hand.

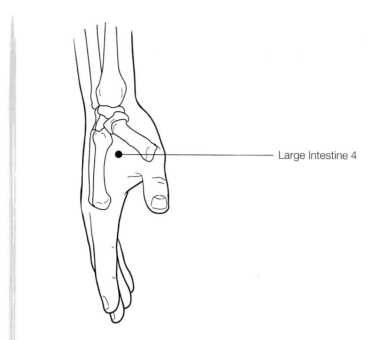

Large Intestine 4

Benefits: Relieves tension, pain and cramping in the hand and fingers.

Note: If pregnant, see pp. 10–11.

For aching and tired muscles in the legs, add the following acupoints:

Urinary Bladder 40

Location: At the back of the knee, between the tendons.

Technique: Bend the knees slightly and place the thumbs at the side of the kneecaps for support and the fingers behind the knees. Locate the point with the index or middle fingers, feeling gently for the hollow in between the tendons. Do not press on the tendons themselves and avoid any varicose veins.

Benefits: Improves circulation and relieves tiredness in the legs.

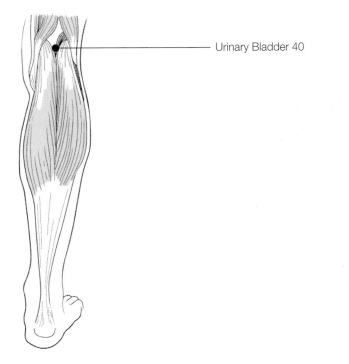

Urinary Bladder 40

Urinary Bladder 60

Location: In the depression behind the ankle bone on the outside edge of the ankle.

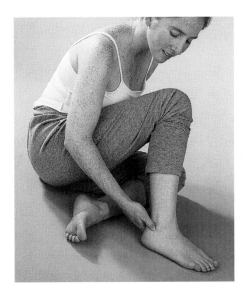

Technique: Place the right hand behind the right leg. Rest the fingers on the inside of the ankle for support and locate the acupoint on the outside edge of the ankle, using the thumb. Apply acupressure with the thumb angled slightly downwards towards the sole of the foot. Alternatively, if it is more comfortable, rest the thumb on the inside ankle and apply pressure with the index or middle finger. Repeat on other ankle.

Benefits: Relieves aching in the lower legs and pain in the heels.

Note: If pregnant, see pp. 10–11.

Stomach 36

Location: Four finger widths below the kneecap on the outside edge of the leg bone (tibia).

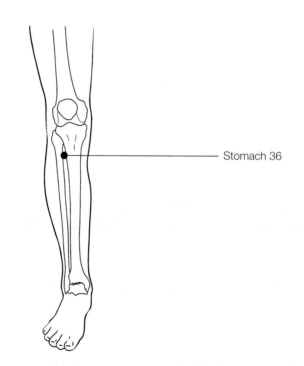

Stomach 36

Technique: Place fingers behind leg for support and locate acupoint with thumb. Apply acupressure angled slightly downwards towards the foot. Repeat for other leg.

Benefits: Promotes circulation, increases energy in the whole body and relieves tiredness in the legs.

Kidney 1

Location: A third of the way down the sole of the foot, in the depression just below the ball of the foot.

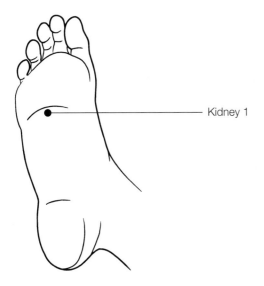

Kidney 1

Technique: Turn the sole of the foot upwards or sideways and support the foot with the fingers. Apply pressure perpendicularly, using one or both thumbs, one on top of the other. Repeat on other foot.

Benefits: Increases general vitality and relieves aching and pain in the legs.

JOINT PROBLEMS

Bone health and strength can be maintained using the general acupressure point *Urinary Bladder 62* (see pp. 233–4) combined with regular gentle exercise of all the joints and supporting muscles and tendons and careful diet. Arthritic pain may be eased by cutting down on acidic foods such as red meat and coffee, also citrus fruits, dairy products and plants from the nightshade family (*Solanaceae*), such as potatoes and tomatoes. Eating plenty of leafy green vegetables and fish, sunflower, linseed or wheatgerm oils may also help. Supplements of Evening Primrose Oil, Green-lipped Mussel and Devil's Claw have given many relief, but epileptics should not use Evening Primrose Oil without medical supervision.

Pain relief and increased flexibility of individual joints can be obtained using local acupressure points (see Chapter 2, The Joints, pp. 109–34). However, when rheumatism or arthritis affects joints throughout the body or moves from one joint to another, the following points may be added:

Governor Vessel 14

Location: At the back of the neck, between the seventh cervical vertebra and the first thoracic vertebra, approximately level with the shoulder.

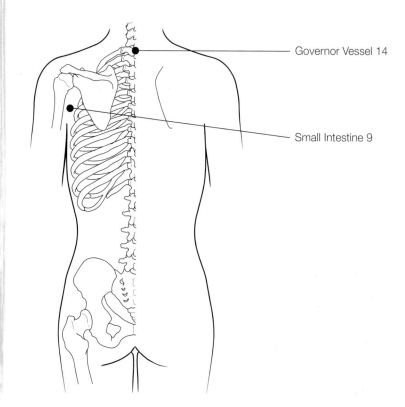

Governor Vessel 14

Small Intestine 9

Technique: Place one hand behind the neck and locate the point with the middle or index finger. Apply acupressure perpendicularly in the slight hollow between the vertebral joints.

Benefits: Strengthens the bones in the neck, shoulders and upper back; relieves pain.

Small Intestine 9

Location: Below the shoulder just above the crease when the arms are at the sides.

Technique: Place one arm at the side of the body and stretch the opposite hand around behind the shoulder. Locate point with middle finger and apply acupressure angled upwards towards the shoulder blade. Repeat behind other shoulder.

Benefits: Increases mobility in the hand, arm and shoulder; relieves pain and swelling.

Gall Bladder 30

Location: On the side of the buttock in the depression underneath the thigh bone and two thirds of the distance between the tip of the sacrum and the crest of the hip.

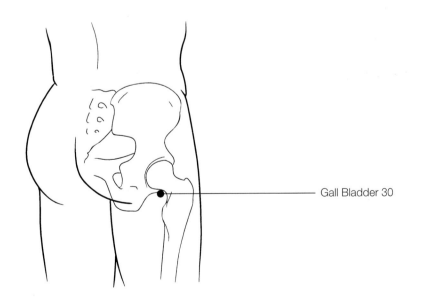

Gall Bladder 30

Technique: Locate this point lying on your side with the thigh raised. Press into the point firmly with either the middle or index finger or the knuckle. Roll over onto the other side and repeat.

Benefits: Increases mobility and relieves pain in the hip joint and legs.

Stomach 34

Location: Three finger widths above the kneecap in the depression on the outer edge of the muscle.

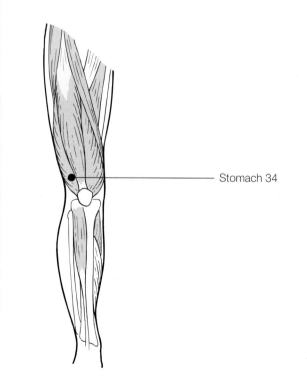

Stomach 34

Technique: Support knee with the fingers and locate acupoint with the thumb. Apply acupressure angled slightly downwards towards the knee. Repeat on other leg.

Benefits: Improves mobility in the knee joint and lower legs and relieves pain and swelling of the knee.

Small Intestine 3

Location: In the depression underneath the knuckle of the little finger in line with the crease when a loose fist is made.

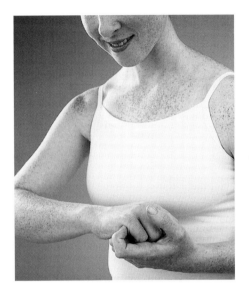

Technique: Curl the fingers of one hand over the fingers of the opposite hand for support. Locate the point using the nail of the index finger and apply acupressure angled inwards underneath the bone. Repeat on other hand.

Benefits: Reduces general aching in the body and relieves stiffness and pain in the neck, back, wrist and fingers.

Urinary Bladder 62

Location: On the outside of the ankle in the depression directly below the tip of the ankle bone.

Technique: Place the fingers around the back of the ankle for support and locate the acupoint with the thumb. Apply acupressure angled slightly downwards towards the little toe. Repeat on other foot.

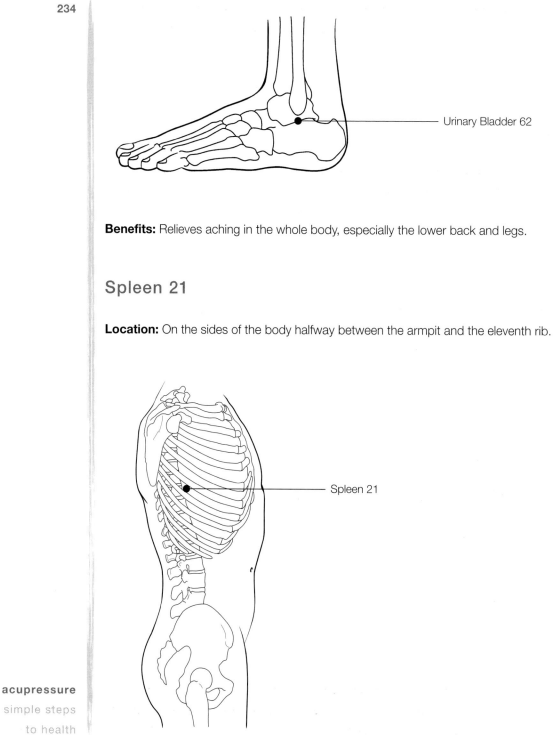

Urinary Bladder 62

Benefits: Relieves aching in the whole body, especially the lower back and legs.

Spleen 21

Location: On the sides of the body halfway between the armpit and the eleventh rib.

Spleen 21

Technique: Cross the arm over the front of the body and locate the acupoint using the middle or index finger. Apply acupressure angled perpendicularly. Repeat on other side using opposite arm.

Benefits: Relieves general aching and weakness in the body.

ALLERGIES

Allergies can be prevented or eased by ensuring a strong and healthy liver and digestive organs, by strengthening the lungs and clearing the airways, and by building immunity (see pp. 238–44). Useful acupoints for achieving this are:

Large Intestine 4

Location: In the centre of the triangle made by the bones of the thumb and the fingers. Can also be located at the end of the crease made by the index finger and thumb when they are pressed together.

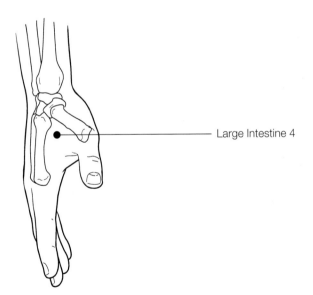

Large Intestine 4

Technique: Support the palm of the left hand in the fingers of the right hand and locate the acupoint with the right thumb. Apply acupressure, angling the thumb slightly towards the wrist. Repeat for other hand.

Benefits: Strengthens the large intestine, relieves allergic reactions and eases symptoms in the face and upper body.

Note: If pregnant, see pp. 10–11.

Triple Heater 5

Location: On the outside of the forearm 3 finger widths above the wrist in the depression between the arm bones (radius and ulna).

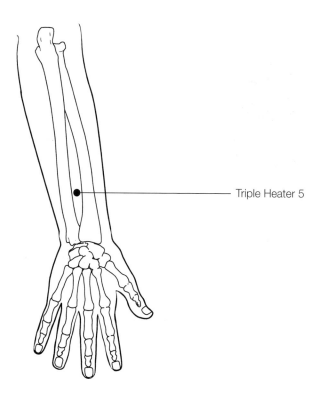

Triple Heater 5

Technique: Measure 3 finger widths from the wrist with the opposite hand. Locate the point with the index finger and support directly underneath the arm with the thumb or use the thumb to apply pressure and support with the fingers. Apply acupressure perpendicularly downwards. Repeat for other arm.

Benefits: Improves the circulation and decreases allergic reactions.

Liver 3

Location: On the top of the foot in the web between the first and second toes, just before the join of the small bones of the foot.

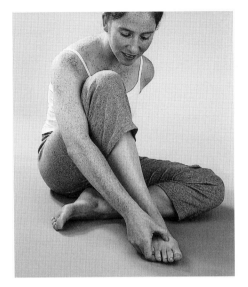

Technique: Place the fingers under the foot for support and press into the point perpendicularly with the thumb. Take care to apply pressure in the hollow between the bone and the tendons rather than on the tendons or blood vessels themselves. Repeat for other foot.

Benefits: Strengthens the liver and reduces allergic sensitivity.

Stomach 36

Location: Four finger widths below the kneecap on the outside edge of the leg bone (tibia).

Technique: Place fingers behind leg for support and locate acupoint with thumb. Apply acupressure angled slightly downwards towards the foot. Repeat on other leg.

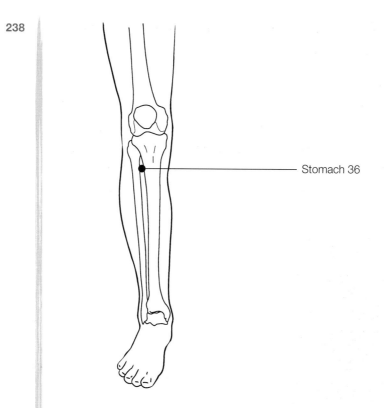

Stomach 36

Benefits: Increases vitality and resistance to allergens.

See also Sinusitis, Nasal Catarrh and Hay Fever (pp. 96–7), Eye Problems (pp. 86–8), Headaches and Migraine (pp. 59–70) and Skin Problems (pp. 219–23).

THE IMMUNE SYSTEM

Acupressure is very effective in helping to boost immunity, alongside healthy diet, exercise and adequate rest. It can also help to relieve symptoms and promote well-being in immune deficiency disorders such as Chronic Fatigue Syndrome and AIDS.

Breathing exercises, posture, balanced exercises and relaxed environment are also important. Daily intake of vitamin C is essential, especially when you feel run down and fatigued. Good sources are kiwi fruit and rosehips. If using supplements, a buffered form such as calcium ascorbate is more easily digested; decrease the dosage if stools become loose.

Acupoints for boosting the immune system, which should be used on a daily ongoing basis for immune deficiency disorders, are as follows:

Governor Vessel 20

Location: At the top of the head on the midline between the tops of the 2 ears and in line with the top of the nose. Locate the point by placing the thumbs on the top of each ear and stretching the middle fingers out to meet at the top of the head.

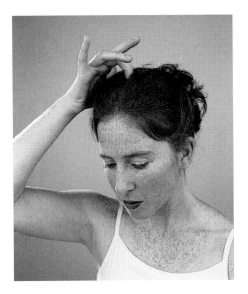

Technique: Apply acupressure perpendicularly into the scalp, using the middle or index fingertip of one hand. For firmer pressure, rest the middle or index fingertip of the other hand on top of the nail of this finger and apply gentle pressure with both fingers simultaneously. The point should be felt as a small depression in the scalp and may feel slightly tender. **Do not overstimulate this point if you have high blood pressure.**

Benefits: Boosts energy in the body and stimulates the immune system.

Governor Vessel 4

Location: On the spine, in the depression between the second and third lumbar vertebrae, approximately level with the waist.

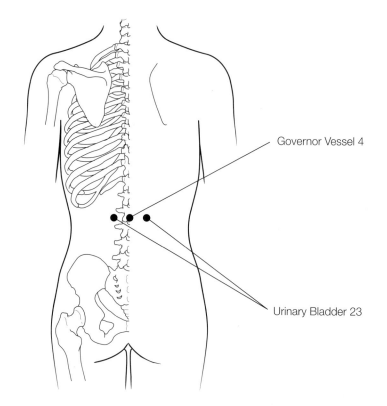

Governor Vessel 4

Urinary Bladder 23

Technique: Place the thumb around the waist and use the middle finger to locate the point. Apply pressure gently in the space between the vertebrae.

Benefits: Strengthens the kidneys and the immune system; boosts vitality.

Urinary Bladder 23

Location: On the lower back 2 finger widths on either side of the spine, approximately level with the waist, by the lower edge of the second lumbar vertebra.

Technique: Place the thumbs on either side of the waist and locate the point on both sides of the spine using the middle fingers. Alternatively, lie on the floor and, arching the back slightly, place two tennis balls level with the points and then gently lower the back onto them.

Benefits: Strengthens the kidneys and the immune system; boosts vitality.

Large Intestine 4

Location: In the centre of the triangle made by the bones of the thumb and the fingers. Can also be located at the end of the crease made by the index finger and thumb when they are pressed together.

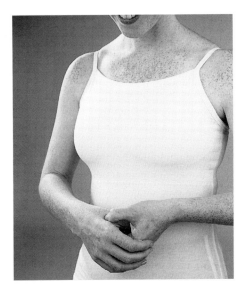

Technique: Support the palm of the left hand in the fingers of the right hand and locate the acupoint with the right thumb. Apply acupressure, angling the thumb slightly towards the wrist. Repeat for other hand.

Benefits: Improves immune response and strengthens the upper body.

Note: If pregnant, see pp. 10–11.

Stomach 36

Location: Four finger widths below the kneecap on the outside edge of the leg bone (tibia).

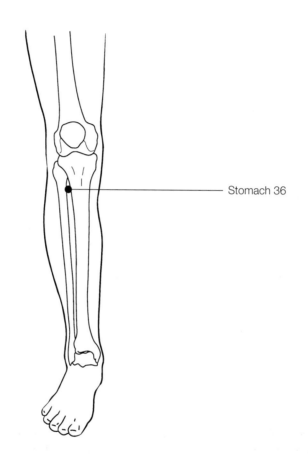

Stomach 36

Technique: Place the fingers behind the leg for support and locate the acupoint with the thumb. Apply acupressure angled slightly downwards towards the foot. Repeat for other leg.

Benefits: Increases vitality, strengthens the digestive organs and boosts immunity.

Conception Vessel 6

Location: Two finger widths below the navel on the midline of the abdomen.

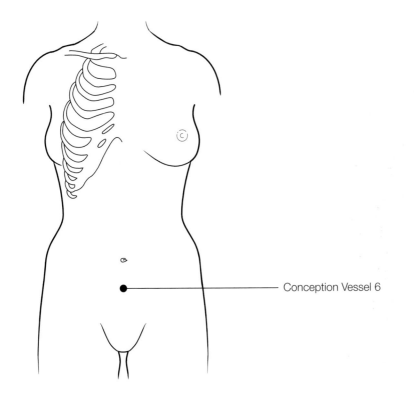

Conception Vessel 6

Technique: Place 2 fingers of one hand horizontally below the navel and locate the point using the middle or index finger of the other hand. Apply pressure perpendicularly and use gentle rotating movements with the fingertip.

Benefits: Increases vitality and strengthens immunity.

Liver 3

Location: On the top of the foot in the web between the first and second toes, just before the join of the small bones of the foot.

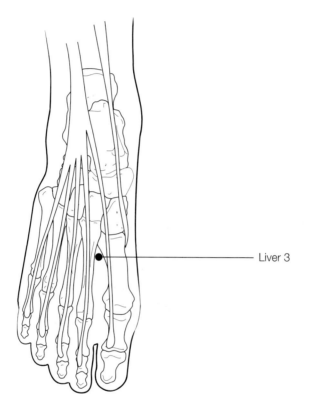

Liver 3

Technique: Place the fingers under the foot for support and press into the point perpendicularly with the thumb. Take care to apply pressure in the hollow between the bone and the tendons rather than on the tendons or blood vessels themselves. Repeat for other foot.

Benefits: Strengthens the liver, overcomes the effects of exercise, stress, strain and toxins in the body.

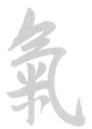

Mental and Emotional Health

Oriental medicine views physical and meridian balance as an important aspect of mental and emotional health since the mind and body are believed to be closely connected. Acupressure points that strengthen the internal organs and promote circulation through the vessels and meridians therefore also help maintain mental and emotional balance:

Governor Vessel 20

Location: At the top of the head on the midline between the tops of the 2 ears and in line with the top of the nose. Locate the point by placing the thumbs on the top of each ear and stretching the middle fingers out to meet at the top of the head.

Technique: Apply acupressure perpendicularly into the scalp, using the middle or index fingertip of one hand. For firmer pressure you can rest the middle or index fingertip of the other hand on top of the nail of the finger locating the point and apply gentle pressure with both fingers simultaneously. The point should be felt as a small depression in the scalp and may feel slightly tender. **Do not overstimulate this point if suffering from high blood pressure.**

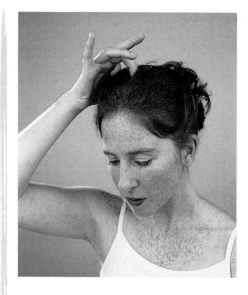

Benefits: Increases mental alertness and concentration and balances the mind.

Large Intestine 4

Location: In the centre of the triangle made by the bones of the thumb and the fingers. Can also be located at the end of the crease made by the index finger and thumb when they are pressed together.

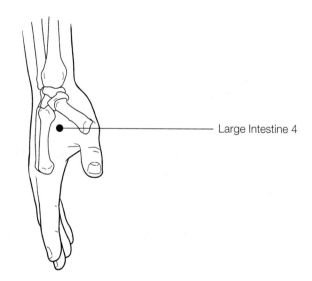

Large Intestine 4

Technique: Support the palm of the left hand in the fingers of the right hand and locate the acupoint with the right thumb. Apply acupressure, angling the thumb slightly towards the wrist. Repeat on other hand.

Benefits: Clears the meridian channels in the upper body and enhances mental function. Can relieve worry and anxiety.

Note: If pregnant, see pp. 10–11.

Heart 7

Location: On the outside edge of the wrist crease closest to the palm, in the hollow in line with the little finger.

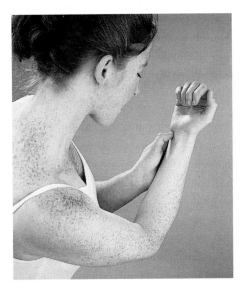

Technique: Turn the palm upwards and support the wrist in the fingers of the opposite hand. Locate the point with the thumb and apply pressure angled downwards towards the little finger. Repeat for other wrist.

Benefits: Calms the heart and mind. A key point for any kind of worry and anxiety or sleep disturbance.

Pericardium 6

Location: Between the tendons on the inside of the arm, 3 finger widths above the wrist crease closest to the palm.

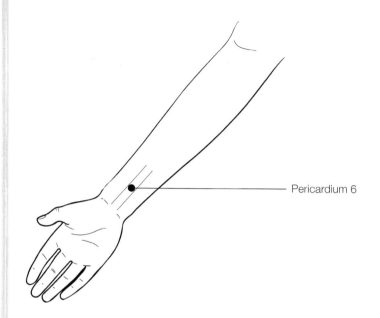

Pericardium 6

Technique: Measure up from the wrist crease to locate the point. Support the wrist with the fingers of the opposite hand and apply acupressure to the point using the thumb, angled downwards towards the middle finger. Repeat for other arm.

Benefits: Calms the mind and relieves anxiety.

Mental and Emotional Problems

Acupressure can help to relieve common mental and emotional problems, including anxiety, poor memory and concentration, irritability, depression and insomnia.

ANXIETY

Use the general mental health acupoints whenever you feel anxiety growing inside you; don't wait till you are a nervous wreck or in a state of panic! The earlier you can use the points the more equipped you will be to deal with whatever is causing your anxiety.

Repeat on an hourly basis and keep using on a daily basis until the crisis is completely over. The heart and digestive organs have a powerful influence on the mind and emotions respectively, so adding the following acupoints can help:

Conception Vessel 6

Location: Two finger widths below the navel on the midline of the abdomen.

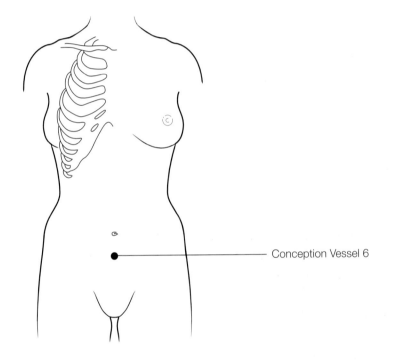

Conception Vessel 6

Technique: Place 2 fingers of one hand horizontally below the navel and locate the point using the middle or index finger of the other hand. Apply pressure perpendicularly and use gentle rotating movements with the fingertip.

Benefits: Strengthens vital energy and increases the ability to cope.

Note: If pregnant see pp. 10–11.

Conception Vessel 12

Location: On the midline of the abdomen, halfway between the navel and the edge of the breast bone.

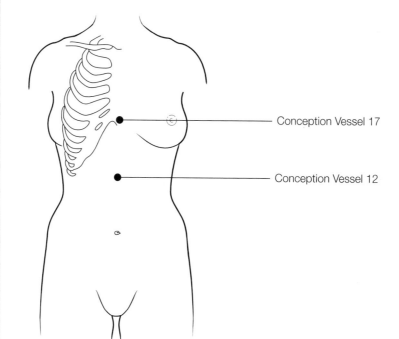

Conception Vessel 17

Conception Vessel 12

Technique: Apply acupressure perpendicularly, using either the index or middle finger.

Benefits: Balances the digestive organs and helps to restore emotional stability.

Conception Vessel 17

Location: In the middle of the chest, in line with the nipples.

Technique: Locate the point with the middle or index finger and apply pressure perpendicularly against the breastbone, using gentle rotating movements.

Benefits: Calms the heart and mind.

Stomach 36

Location: Four finger widths below the kneecap on the outside edge of the leg bone (tibia).

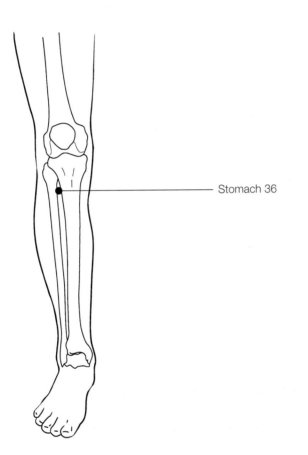

Stomach 36

Technique: Place fingers behind the leg for support and locate acupoint with the thumb. Apply acupressure angled slightly downwards towards foot. Repeat on other leg.

Benefits: Invigorates the digestive organs and increases vitality and emotional stability.

Thought to be related to kidney function, which can be impaired by excessive stress, strain and/or fatigue, poor memory and concentration can be enhanced by adding:

Urinary Bladder 10

Location: On the nape of the neck, just inside the hairline, 2 finger widths on either side of the spine in the depression on the side of the large neck muscle (trapezius).

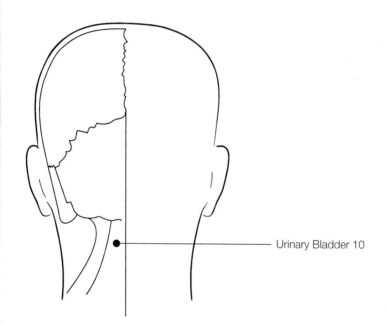

Urinary Bladder 10

Technique: Rest the fingers on the back of the scalp. Locate the acupoint with the thumbs and apply pressure perpendicularly to the base of the skull, on either side of the spine.

Benefits: Relieves tension and increases circulation in the neck and head. Improves memory and concentration.

Urinary Bladder 23

Location: On the lower back 2 finger widths on either side of the spine, approximately level with the waist, by the lower edge of the second lumbar vertebra.

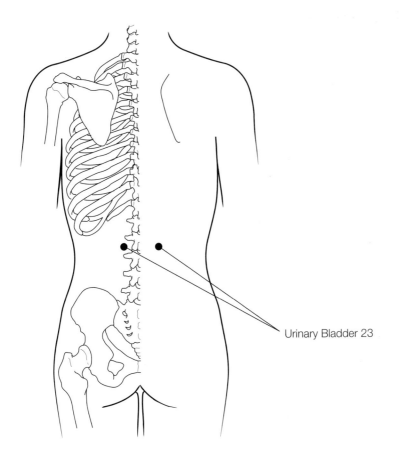

Urinary Bladder 23

Technique: Place the thumbs on either side of the waist and locate the point on both sides of the spine using the middle fingers. Alternatively, lie on the floor and, arching the back slightly, place the knuckles or two tennis balls level with the points and then gently lower the back onto them.

Benefits: Strengthens the kidneys, which are said to have a powerful effect on memory and concentration.

Kidney 6

Location: On the inside of the ankle, 1 thumb width below the tip of the ankle bone.

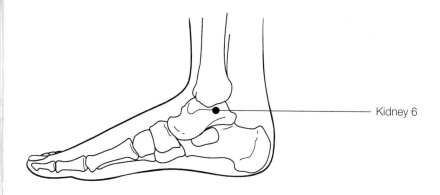

Kidney 6

Technique: Place the fingers over the top of the ankle for support and apply acupressure perpendicularly with the thumb. Repeat on other foot.

Benefits: Helps to clear the mind and improve concentration.

IRRITABILITY

In Oriental medicine chronic irritability is related to liver imbalance. Adding the following points on a daily basis is useful:

Urinary Bladder 18

Location: Two finger widths on either side of the spine, level with the ninth thoracic vertebra.

Technique: Lie on the floor with the knees bent and place either the knuckles or two tennis balls under the back level with the point. Gradually lower the weight of the back onto the knuckles or balls to apply acupressure to the point.

Benefits: Improves liver function and reduces irritability.

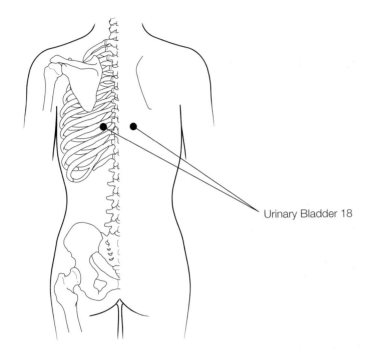

Urinary Bladder 18

Liver 3

Location: On the top of the foot in the web between the first and second toes, just before the join of the small bones of the foot.

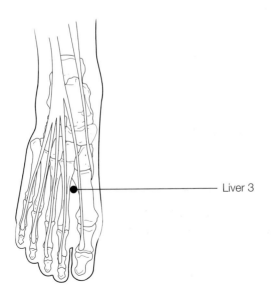

Liver 3

Technique: Place the fingers under the foot for support and press into the point perpendicularly with the thumb. Take care to apply pressure in the hollow between the bone and the tendons rather than on the tendons or blood vessels themselves. Repeat on other foot.

Benefits: Improves liver function and reduces irritability.

DEPRESSION

This can be related to poor circulation to the head or imbalance in the liver, stomach or spleen as well as to poor diet, lack of exercise, lack of exposure to sunlight and emotional problems. Add the following points:

Governor Vessel 26

Location: In the groove below the nose, slightly more than halfway up.

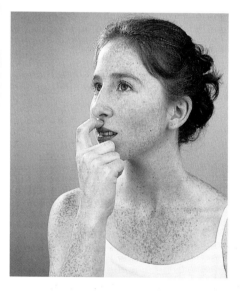

Technique: Locate the point with the nail edge or fingertip of the index or middle finger and place the thumb under the chin for support. Apply acupressure lightly, pressing perpendicularly against the gums underneath.

Caution: Do not overstimulate this point if you have high blood pressure; stop immediately if you feel unwell or uncomfortable.

Benefits: Clears the mind and relieves depression.

Urinary Bladder 10

Location: On the nape of the neck, just inside the hairline, 2 finger widths on either side of the spine in the depression on the side of the large neck muscle (trapezius).

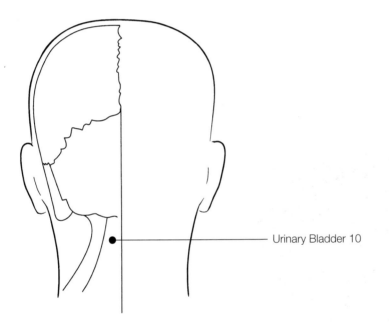

Urinary Bladder 10

Technique: Rest fingers on the back of the scalp. Locate acupoint with the thumbs and apply pressure perpendicularly to base of the skull, on either side of the spine.

Benefits: Improves circulation in the neck and head and can relieve depression.

Conception Vessel 12

Location: On the midline of the abdomen, halfway between the navel and the edge of the breast bone.

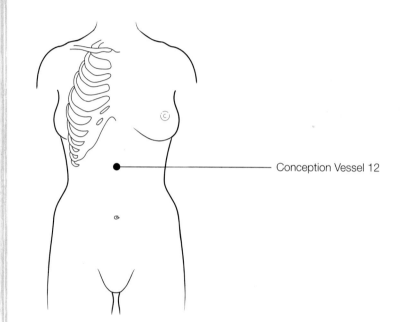

Conception Vessel 12

Technique: Apply acupressure perpendicularly, using either the index or middle finger.

Benefits: Balances the digestive organs and improves sense of well-being.

Liver 3

Location: On the top of the foot in the web between the first and second toes, just before the join of the small bones of the foot.

Technique: Place the fingers under the foot for support and press into the point perpendicularly with the thumb. Take care to apply pressure in the hollow between the bone and the tendons rather than on the tendons or blood vessels themselves. Repeat for other foot.

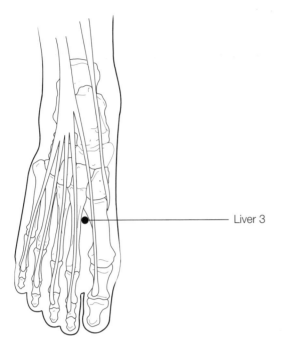

Liver 3

Benefits: Improves liver function and relieves depression.

INSOMNIA

Insomnia can be relieved by calming the heart and mind, so the mental health acupoints *Heart 7* and *Pericardium 6*, which have this function, are especially important. Add the following:

Gall Bladder 12

Location: Behind the ears in the depression under the bone (mastoid).

Technique: Place fingers on the back of the head and locate point with the thumbs. Apply acupressure angled slightly upwards under the bone on both sides of the head.

Benefits: Reduces restlessness, disturbed sleep and excessive dreaming due to liver imbalance.

Gall Bladder 12

Spleen 6

Location: On the inside of the leg, 4 finger widths above the tip of the ankle bone and just inside the bone of the leg (tibia).

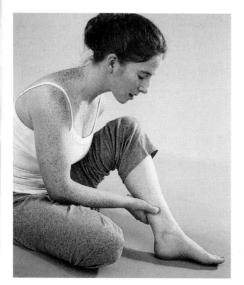

Technique: Measure 4 finger widths up from the ankle bone with one hand and then use the thumb of the other hand to locate the acupoint. Apply acupressure perpendicularly. Repeat on other leg.

Benefits: Balances and strengthens the liver, spleen and kidneys and nourishes the blood, making sleep easier and calmer.

Note: If pregnant, see pp. 10–11.

Kidney 3

Location: On the inside of the ankle in the depression level with the tip of the ankle bone.

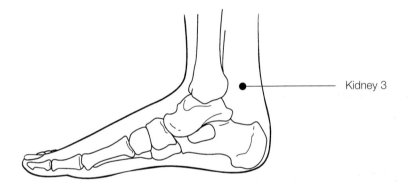

Kidney 3

Technique: Place fingers of the opposite hand behind the ankle for support and locate point with the thumb. Apply pressure perpendicularly or use small rotations. Repeat for other foot.

Benefits: Improves kidney and heart function, making sleep easier and more peaceful.

HYPERACTIVITY

This condition, typified by extreme restlessness, irritability, poor concentration and sometimes violence, can be related to severe forms of food allergy, especially in young children. Allergy testing is therefore a good idea (see Useful Addresses). Essential fatty acid deficiency may also be a factor. Acupressure may help to restore digestive balance and mental and physical calm in the body. In conjunction with dietary change, use the general mental health points and add the following:

Pericardium 8

Location: In the middle of the palm between the bones leading to the index and middle fingers. Can also be located by bending the middle finger inwards until it touches the palm.

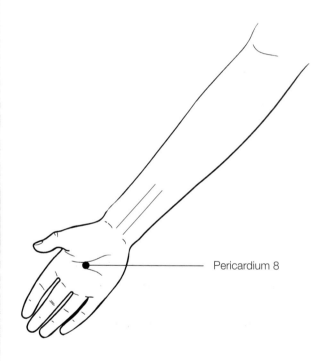

Pericardium 8

Technique: Support the palm with the fingers of the opposite hand and locate the acupoint with the thumb. Apply acupressure angled slightly towards the middle finger. Repeat on opposite palm.

Benefits: Calms the mind and reduces mental agitation.

Lung 11

Location: On the outside edge of the thumb, by the corner of the thumbnail.

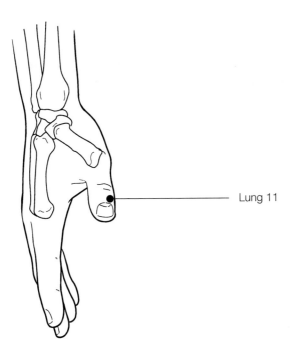

Lung 11

Technique: Support the thumb in the fingers of the opposite hand and apply acupressure using the nail of the opposite thumb. Repeat on other hand.

Benefits: Very effective in calming agitation and restoring mental clarity.

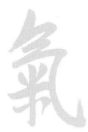

Healthy Pregnancy

Acupressure can safely be used during pregnancy as long as only light pressure is applied and particular caution is taken over the points that are used for labour and delivery, which stimulate uterine contractions. These points are clearly marked in the text and should simply be touched and 'held' while you concentrate on breathing and visualization, rather than stimulated by pressure.

Preconceptual Care and Healthy Pregnancy

A healthy pregnancy begins with preconceptual care in the form of exercise, building vitality, strengthening the organs and muscles that will support pregnancy, creating good nutritional balance and mental and emotional preparedness. Essential nutrients are folic acid, zinc, iron, calcium, magnesium, vitamin C, the B vitamins and essential fatty acids (EFAs). Acupressure points that strengthen the kidneys, liver, spleen, uterus and abdominal muscles are all important before conception and during pregnancy. A good preconceptual acupressure routine that can be used up to 6 months before attempting conception is given below. The same points can be used during pregnancy to maintain good health, but pressure should be much lighter and always comfortable.

Governor Vessel 23

Location: About 1 finger width inside the hairline on the midline of the scalp in line with the top of the nose.

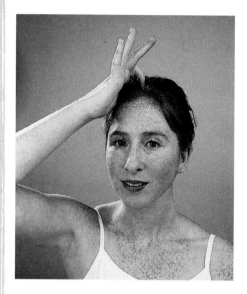

Technique: Apply acupressure perpendicularly, using the middle or index fingertip. Rest the thumb on the temple at the side of the head for support.

Benefits: Tones the uterus, increases vitality and helps to balance the hormonal system.

Urinary Bladder 23

Location: On the lower back 2 finger widths on either side of the spine, approximately level with the waist, by the lower edge of the second lumbar vertebra.

Technique: Place the thumbs on either side of the waist and locate the point on both sides of the spine using the middle fingers. Alternatively, lie on the floor and, arching the back slightly, place the knuckles or two tennis balls level with the points and then gently lower the back onto them.

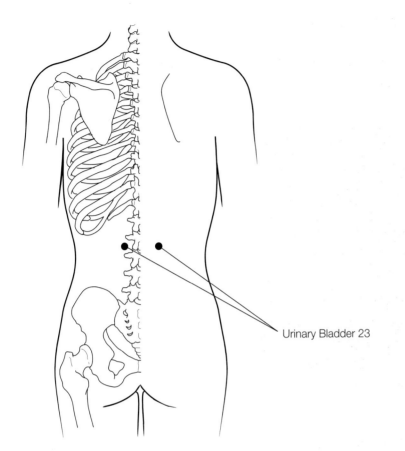

Urinary Bladder 23

Benefits: Strengthens the kidneys and aids fertility.

Conception Vessel 6

Location: Two finger widths below the navel on the midline of the abdomen.

Technique: Place 2 fingers of one hand horizontally below the navel and locate the point using the middle or index finger of the other hand. Apply gentle pressure perpendicularly and use light rotating movements with the fingertip.

Benefits: Increases vitality, tones the abdominal muscles and organs, and gives strength to the reproductive organs.

Conception Vessel 6

Stomach 36

Location: Four finger widths below the kneecap on the outside edge of the leg bone (tibia).

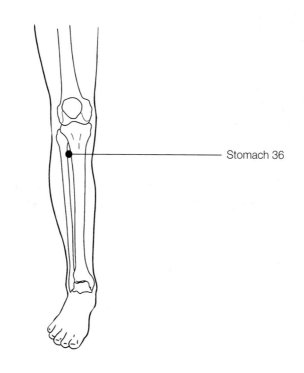

Stomach 36

Technique: Place fingers behind the leg for support and locate acupoint with the thumb. Apply acupressure angled slightly downwards towards foot. Repeat for other leg.

Benefits: General tonic point that increases vitality in the body as a whole and strengthens the spleen and stomach.

Kidney 3

Location: On the inside of the ankle in the depression level with the tip of the ankle bone.

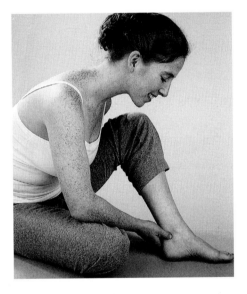

Technique: Place fingers of the opposite hand behind the ankle for support and locate point with thumb. Apply pressure perpendicularly or use small rotations. Repeat on other ankle.

Benefits: Strengthens the kidneys and aids fertility.

Pregnancy Problems

Acupressure is very effective in relieving many of the minor discomforts associated with pregnancy.

MORNING SICKNESS

Apply acupressure to the following point every morning before you get out of bed and use at any time during the day when you feel nauseous. Alternatively, use acupressure wristbands to maintain pressure day and night.

Pericardium 6

Location: Between the tendons on the inside of the arm, 3 finger widths above the wrist crease closest to the palm.

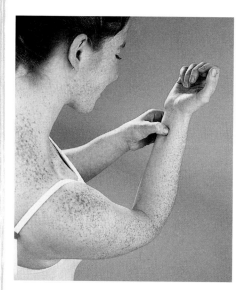

Technique: Measure up from the wrist crease to locate the point. Support the wrist with the fingers of the opposite hand and apply acupressure to the point using the thumb, angled downwards towards the middle finger. Repeat on opposite wrist.

Benefits: Relieves morning sickness, nausea and travel sickness.

LOW BACK PAIN

See The Back (pp. 120–26).

ACHING LEGS AND VARICOSE VEINS

As well as adding the following points, make sure to sit or lie with the legs raised several times during the day, especially in the evening before going to bed. See also Varicose Veins (pp. 159–60).

Stomach 36

Location: Four finger widths below the kneecap on the outside edge of the leg bone (tibia).

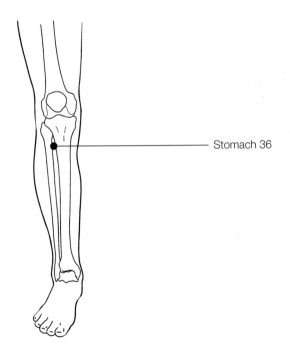

Stomach 36

Technique: Place the fingers behind the leg for support with the thumb. Apply acupressure angled slightly downwards towards the foot. Repeat for other leg.

Benefits: Increases circulation in the legs and relieves tiredness.

Liver 3

Location: On the top of the foot in the web between the first and second toes, just before the join of the small bones of the foot.

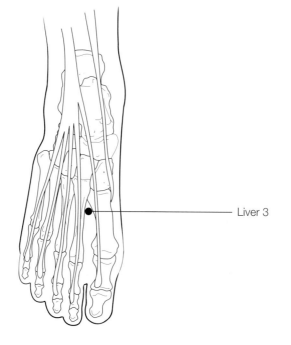

Liver 3

Technique: Place fingers under foot for support and press into point perpendicularly with thumb. Take care to apply pressure in the hollow between the bone and the tendons rather than on the tendons or blood vessels themselves. Repeat on other foot.

Benefits: Increases circulation in the legs, relieves muscular aching and helps to prevent varicose veins.

WATER RETENTION (OEDEMA)

Urinary Bladder 23

Location: On the lower back 2 finger widths on either side of the spine, approximately level with the waist, by the lower edge of the second lumbar vertebra.

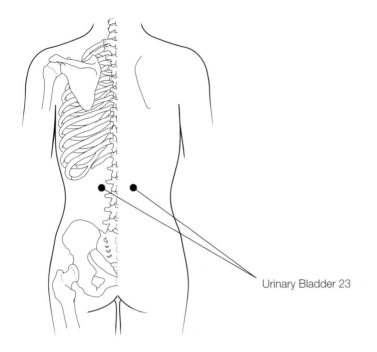

Urinary Bladder 23

Technique: Place the thumbs on either side of the waist and locate the point on both sides of the spine using the middle fingers. Alternatively, lie on the floor and, arching the back slightly, place the knuckles or two tennis balls level with the points and then gently lower the back onto them.

Benefits: Stimulates the kidneys and the elimination of excess water from the body.

Kidney 3

Location: On the inside of the ankle in the depression level with the tip of the ankle bone.

Technique: Place fingers of the opposite hand behind the ankle for support and locate point with the thumb. Apply pressure perpendicularly or use small rotations. Repeat on other ankle.

Benefits: Reduces swelling in the ankles and promotes the release of excess fluids in the lower limbs.

See also Water Retention and Swelling (Oedema) (pp. 184–7).

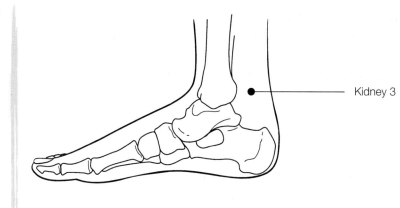

Kidney 3

BREAST TENDERNESS

Stomach 16

Location: At the top of the breasts in line with the nipple, between the third and fourth ribs.

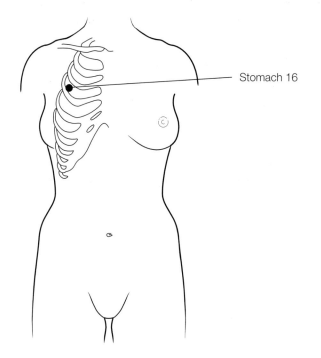

Stomach 16

Technique: Place the thumbs in the armpits for support and locate the point using the middle or index fingers. Apply acupressure in the space between the ribs.

Benefits: Relieves breast tenderness and pain and improves lactation.

FATIGUE

Acupoints *Stomach 36* and *Conception Vessel 6* (described in the previous section for healthy pregnancy) are especially important and can be used night and morning or at regular intervals throughout the day to relieve fatigue. As pregnancy develops, acupoint *Conception Vessel 6* should only be lightly touched rather than having acupressure applied.

See also Blood Pressure (pp. 157–8).

Healthy Labour and Birth

Acupressure can be very helpful during labour and delivery and can be used to increase the effectiveness of uterine contractions, reduce the time spent in labour and reduce labour pain. It can be applied by a partner, birth attendant or midwife, but point location should be practised beforehand so that application can be swift and easy during labour. Acupressure and massage around the sacrum at the base of the spine can also be effective in inducing labour and help relieve labour pain. However, individual preference for touch and massage during labour varies enormously.

Certain points may also be used to promote delivery of the placenta after birth; however, consult your acupuncturist on this, as direct acupuncture may produce quicker results at this stage.

Large Intestine 4

Location: In the centre of the triangle made by the bones of the thumb and the fingers. Can also be located at the end of the crease made by the index finger and thumb when they are pressed together.

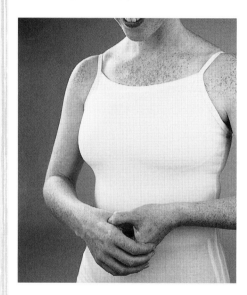

Technique: Support the palm of the left hand in the fingers of the right hand and locate the acupoint with the right thumb. Apply acupressure, angling the thumb slightly towards the wrist. Repeat for other hand.

Benefits: Promotes uterine contractions and relieves labour pain.

Location: On the inside of the leg, 4 finger widths above the tip of the ankle bone and just inside the bone of the leg (tibia).

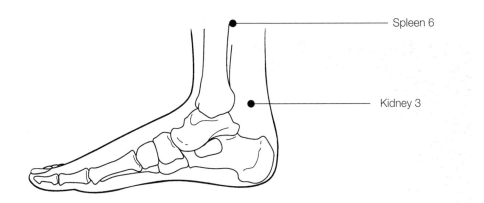

Spleen 6

Kidney 3

Technique: Measure 4 finger widths up from the ankle bone with one hand and then use the thumb of the other hand to locate the acupoint. Apply acupressure perpendicularly. Repeat on other ankle.

Benefits: Strengthens the organs that support and regulate delivery and promotes effective uterine contractions (i.e. contraindicated during pregnancy but effective during labour).

Kidney 3

Location: On the inside of the ankle in the depression level with the tip of the ankle bone.

Technique: Place the fingers of the opposite hand behind the ankle for support and locate the point with the thumb. Apply pressure perpendicularly or use small rotations. Repeat on other ankle.

Benefits: Strengthens the kidneys, reduces fatigue and relieves labour pain.

Urinary Bladder 67

Location: On the outside edge of the little toe at the corner of the toenail.

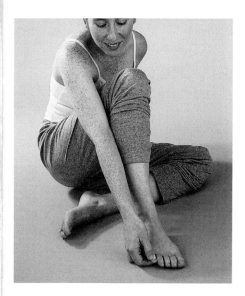

Technique: Support the foot with the fingers and apply acupressure using the nail of the index finger or thumb. Repeat on other foot.

Benefits: Relieves labour pain and promotes uterine contractions. Can also be used for helping to position the baby correctly in the later stages of pregnancy and to turn breech babies. Seek advice from a qualified acupuncturist about this.

Post-Partum Care

Acupressure can be used to rebuild vitality after the birth and to help with lactation and breastfeeding.

Rebuilding Vitality

Use the following points on a daily basis after the birth or ask someone to do them for you. If you have had a Caesarean section, omit *Conception Vessel 6* until the scar is healed. Continue using the points for around 6 weeks or until you feel your energy has been restored. Take rest whenever possible, eat nourishing and wholesome food, and accept all offers of help!

Conception Vessel 6

Location: Two finger widths below the navel on the midline of the abdomen.

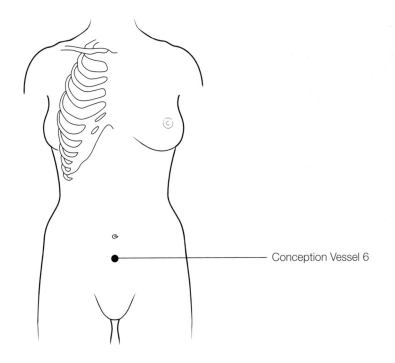

Conception Vessel 6

Technique: Place 2 fingers of one hand horizontally below the navel and locate the point using the middle or index finger of the other hand. Apply pressure perpendicularly and use gentle rotating movements with the fingertip.

Benefits: Helps strengthen the abdominal muscles and revitalize the reproductive organs. Overcomes weakness and fatigue and builds vitality.

Urinary Bladder 23

Location: On the lower back 2 finger widths on either side of the spine, approximately level with the waist, by the lower edge of the second lumbar vertebra.

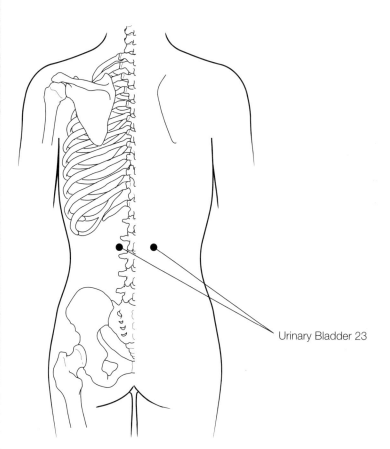

Urinary Bladder 23

Technique: Place the thumbs on either side of the waist and locate the point on both sides of the spine using the middle fingers. Alternatively, lie on the floor and, arching the back slightly, place the knuckles or two tennis balls level with the points and then gently lower the back onto them.

Benefits: Strengthens the kidneys and rebuilds vitality.

Stomach 36

Location: Four finger widths below the kneecap on the outside edge of the leg bone (tibia).

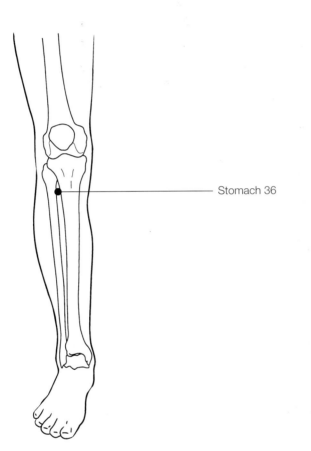

Stomach 36

Technique: Place the fingers behind the leg for support and locate the acupoint with the thumb. Apply acupressure angled slightly downwards towards the foot. Repeat for other leg.

Benefits: Strengthens the abdominal muscles and gynaecological organs and builds vitality.

See also The Immune System (pp. 238–44).

Breastfeeding

The following acupressure points help to increase the production and flow of breast milk, relieve breast and nipple soreness and prevent blocked ducts and mastitis. The application of warm flannels prior to feeding will facilitate milk flow as will a healthy diet rich in essential fatty acids (EFAs) and vitamins and minerals. Good positioning and relaxation help establish comfortable feeding, while gentle massage and alternate hot and cold flannels will help release blocked ducts. Act quickly to prevent mastitis developing, which will then require medical treatment. Cabbage leaves cooled in the fridge and placed inside the bra will ease soreness and swelling and massage with fennel oil will prevent ducts blocking.

Stomach 16

Location: At the top of the breasts in line with the nipples, between the third and fourth ribs.

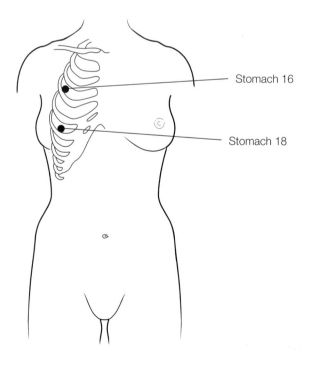

Stomach 16

Stomach 18

Technique: Place the thumbs in the armpits for support and locate the point using the middle or index fingers. Apply acupressure in the space between the ribs.

Benefits: Increases lactation and relieves breast discomfort and pain.

Stomach 18

Location: Just underneath the breast tissue in line with the nipples, in the depression between the fourth and fifth ribs.

Technique: Locate the point with the index or middle finger or the thumb by pressing up gently under the breasts to locate the space between the ribs. Gently apply acupressure between the ribs.

Benefits: Promotes lactation and reduces breast discomfort and pain.

Small Intestine 1

Location: On the outside edge of the little finger by the corner of the fingernail.

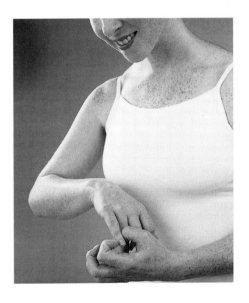

Technique: Support the little finger in the fingers of the opposite hand and apply acupressure with the nail edge of the index or middle finger. Repeat on other hand.

Benefits: Increases the production and flow of breast milk.

See also Vaginal Dryness or Discharge (pp. 206–8), Sexual Health and Vitality (pp. 209–13), Sexual Apathy and Pain (pp. 217–18), Poor Memory and Concentration (pp. 204–6), Depression (pp. 256–9) and Insomnia (pp. 259–61).

part four

Acupressure
First **Aid**

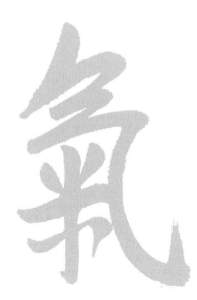

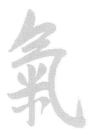

Sometimes we are confronted with an emergency situation where there is no medical help available. At other times a health condition may not require immediate medical attention but prompt action can minimize discomfort and promote a return to well-being. At such moments acupressure is an invaluable tool for minimizing injury and bringing relief. First aid training is offered by many voluntary organizations, so check what is available locally.

First aid acupressure (in alphabetical order) is as follows:

ASTHMA ATTACK

Sit the person down leaning slightly forward and resting on a support such as a table or chair back. Loosen clothing around the throat, ensure a good supply of fresh air and reassure and calm the person. Apply the following acupressure points:

Asthma Relief Acupoint

Location: At the back of the neck 1 finger width on either side of the spine at the junction between the seventh cervical vertebra and the first thoracic vertebra.

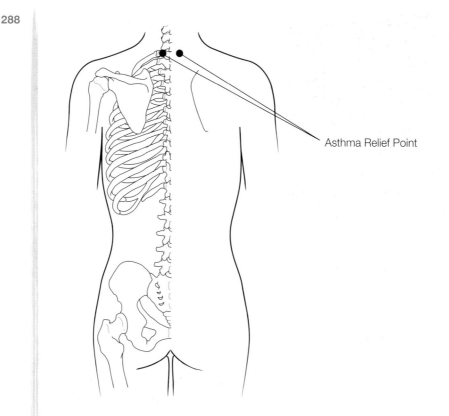

Asthma Relief Point

Technique: Place the hands over the shoulders of the sufferer and locate the point with your thumbs. Apply acupressure firmly in the depression between the two vertebrae. Do not press on the bones themselves.

Benefits: Helps to clear and relax the airways and relieves asthma attacks.

Lung 7

Location: Two finger widths from the wrist crease closest to the palm, on the inside of the forearm, in line with the thumb.

Technique: Support the person's wrist in your hand and locate the point with your thumb. Apply pressure angled down towards the thumb. Repeat on other arm.

Benefits: Helps to strengthen the lungs, open the airways and relieve asthma.

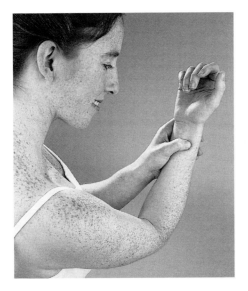

Large Intestine 4

Location: In the centre of the triangle made by the bones of the thumb and the fingers. Can also be located at the end of the crease made by the index finger and thumb when they are pressed together.

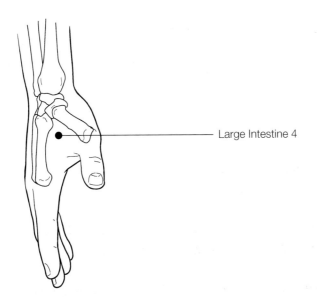

Large Intestine 4

Technique: Support the person's palm in your hand and locate the acupoint with your thumb. Apply acupressure, angling the thumb slightly towards the wrist. Repeat on other hand.

Benefits: Relaxes the upper body and relieves asthma.

Note: If pregnant, see pp. 10–11.

Stomach 40

Location: On the outside edge of the leg bone halfway between the tip of the ankle bone and the middle of the kneecap.

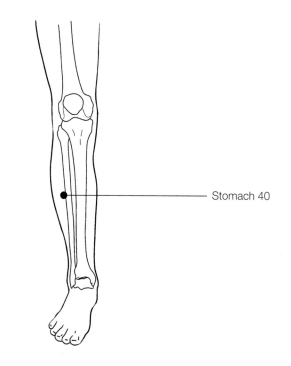

Stomach 40

Technique: Place your hands behind the person's lower legs for support and apply acupressure using your thumbs.

Benefits: Eliminates phlegm and respiratory congestion.

Location: In the depression below the throat, just above the top of the breastbone (sternum).

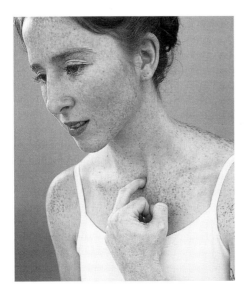

Technique: Locate the point with the middle or index finger of one hand and press in against the bone, not the windpipe.

Benefits: Clears the throat and airways and makes breathing easier.

See also Chapter 4, The Respiratory System (pp. 135–46), including Asthma (pp. 142–5).

ASPHYXIA

If a person has stopped breathing due to suffocation, blockage in the airways, fits, drowning, shock or injury, urgent attention can be life-saving. Call medical assistance immediately and meanwhile loosen clothing, remove any obstruction in the throat, apply mouth-to-mouth resuscitation and use the following emergency acupressure points:

Lung 9

Location: On the wrist crease closest to the palm, on the inside of the wrist in the depression next to the radial artery and in line with the thumb.

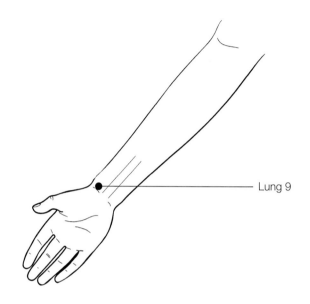

Lung 9

Technique: Support the wrist in your hand with the palm facing upwards. Locate the point with your thumb and apply pressure angled down towards the thumb. Repeat on other arm.

Benefits: Has a direct effect on the lungs and airways, promoting breathing.

Conception Vessel 17

Location: In the middle of the chest, in line with the nipples.

Technique: Locate the point with the middle or index finger of one hand and apply pressure perpendicularly against the breastbone, using gentle rotating movements.

Benefits: Releases obstruction in the chest and promotes breathing.

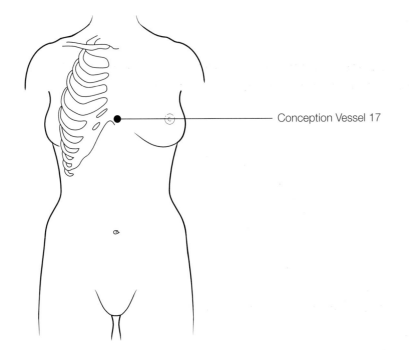

Conception Vessel 17

APPENDICITIS

Characterized by intense local pain in the right-hand lower abdomen, this requires urgent medical attention. Meanwhile apply firm acupressure to the following:

Appendix Acupoint

Location: Approximately 5 thumb widths below the lower edge of the kneecap, located in between the leg bones. Can also be located 3 finger widths below acupoint *Stomach 36*.

Technique: Place your fingers behind the person's leg for support and apply firm perpendicular acupressure with your thumbs.

Benefits: Relieves appendix pain and general pain and swelling in the lower abdomen.

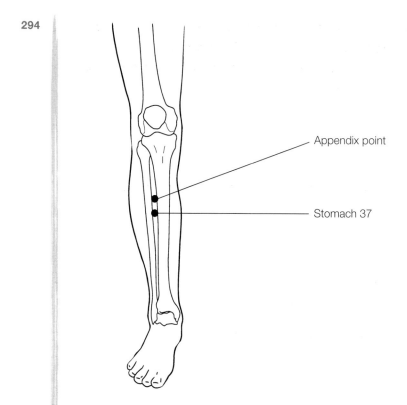

Appendix point

Stomach 37

Stomach 37

Location: Six thumb widths below the kneecap, in between the bones of the leg. Can also be located by placing four fingers of one hand and then four fingers of the other hand down the leg.

Technique: Keeping your fingers behind the person's legs, move your thumbs down from the appendix acupoint and apply firm, perpendicular pressure.

Benefits: Relieves appendix pain and abdominal swelling and regulates large intestine function.

BITES

For animal bites, rinse the wound well with water containing antiseptic, dry it and cover it with a clean dressing. Then seek immediate medical attention in case of infection.

Homoeopathic Arnica can be used to reduce swelling and homoeopathic Hypercal cream will aid healing. Both should be kept on hand at home and are available from homoeopathic pharmacies (see Useful Addresses). For superficial bites, the following acupressure point can be very helpful:

Kidney 24

Location: In between the third and fourth ribs, three finger widths from the midline of the body.

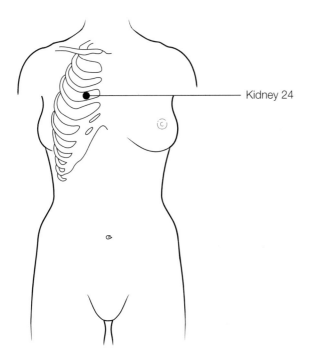

Kidney 24

Technique: Place your fingers under the armpits for support and locate the acupoint using the thumbs. Apply acupressure perpendicularly in the space in between the ribs.

Benefits: Helps to relieve shock, promotes recovery from bites and stings and the elimination of poisons from the body.

BRUISING

Cool the affected area with an ice pack or cold compress. Apply witch hazel or homoeopathic Arnica cream locally as soon as possible. Homoeopathic Arnica tablets can also be taken orally – keep them in the house at all times. Apply the emergency acupressure point:

Large Intestine 15

Location: On the tip of the shoulder in the depression between the bones when the arms are by the sides.

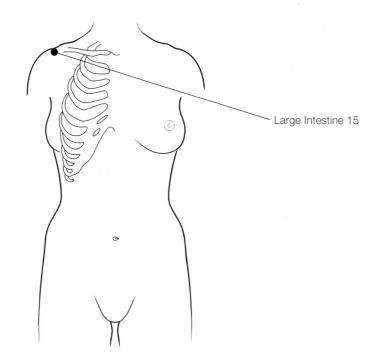

Large Intestine 15

Technique: Place your hands over the person's shoulders and locate the point using your thumbs. Apply acupressure angled slightly upwards towards the shoulder.

Benefits: Emergency acupoint for relieving bruising, swelling and pain, especially in the upper body.

Location: On the top of the foot in the web between the first and second toes, just before the join of the small bones of the foot.

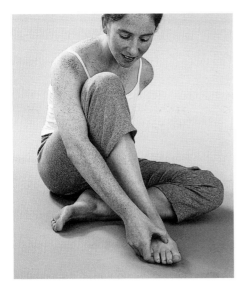

Technique: Place your fingers under both of the person's feet for support and press into the point perpendicularly with your thumbs. Take care to apply pressure in the hollow between the bone and the tendons rather than on the tendons or blood vessels themselves.

Benefits: Promotes repair of small blood vessels and helps to clear bruising.

BURNS

For minor burns, place the injured part in cold water for 5–10 minutes or under a slowly running, cold water tap until pain and heat sensation have completely disappeared. *Never* apply fat or oil such as butter. Healing can be promoted using Calendula cream and the following acupressure points:

Urinary Bladder 65

Location: On the outside edge of the foot in the depression under the bone just beyond the join of the little toe to the foot.

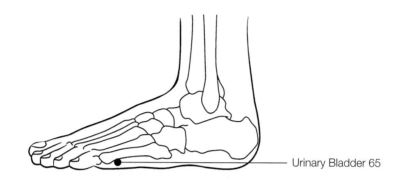

Urinary Bladder 65

Technique: Support the person's feet in your hands and locate the point using your thumbs. Apply acupressure with the nail edge up underneath the bone and angled towards the toe.

Benefits: Helps to relieve pain and promote healing from burns and scalds.

If there is shock, also add the following:

Kidney 1

Location: A third of the way down the sole of the foot, in the depression just below the ball of the foot.

Technique: Turn the sole of the person's foot upwards or sideways and support the foot with the fingers of one hand. Apply pressure perpendicularly, with the thumb of the other hand. Repeat on other foot.

Benefits: Relieves shock and restores energy in the body.

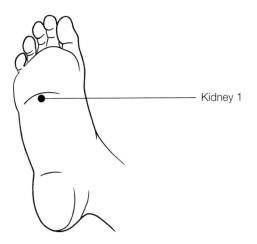

Kidney 1

CRAMPS

Leg cramps may be prevented by regular stretching exercises for the legs and feet and plenty of vitamin E, calcium and magnesium in the diet. To relieve sudden cramps, apply acupressure gently all along the affected muscle. For abdominal cramps see pp. 170–71 and for menstrual cramps and pain, pp. 192–7.

FAINTING

Sit the person down and lean them forward with the head between the knees. Release any tight clothing around the throat and ensure that the person is breathing freely. Apply acupressure as below. To prevent repeated fainting, learn to relax the neck and shoulders, practise breathing exercises and ensure a balanced, nutritious diet with sufficient iron.

Governor Vessel 26

Location: In the groove below the nose, slightly more than halfway up.

Technique: Locate the point with the nail edge or fingertip of the index or middle finger of one hand while cupping the person's chin in your other hand. Apply acupressure lightly, pressing perpendicularly against the gums underneath.

Caution: Do not overstimulate this point if you have high blood pressure; stop immediately if you feel unwell or uncomfortable.

acupressure

first aid

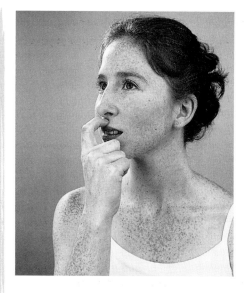

Benefits: Relieves fainting and increases mental alertness.

Pericardium 7

Location: In the middle of the crease nearest the palm on the inside of the wrist between the tendons.

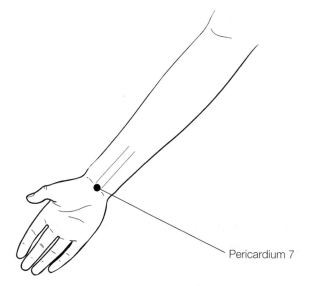

Pericardium 7

Technique: Support the person's wrists in your hands and locate the acupoint with your thumbs. Apply pressure, taking care to press in between the tendons and blood vessels and not on them.

Benefits: Promotes circulation and relieves faintness.

FOOD POISONING

Give the person plenty of fluids and apply the following acupoints:

Large Intestine 4

Location: In the centre of the triangle made by the bones of the thumb and the fingers. Can also be located at the end of the crease made by the index finger and thumb when they are pressed together.

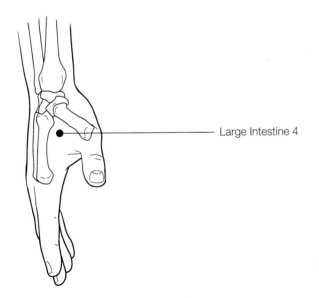

Large Intestine 4

Technique: Support the palm of the person's hand in your hand and locate the acupoint with your thumb. Apply acupressure, angling the thumb slightly towards the wrist. Repeat for other hand.

Benefits: Stimulates the large intestine, promotes elimination and relieves abdominal discomfort.

Note: If pregnant, see pp. 10–11.

Emergency Acupoint for Poisoning

This point can be used in the case of mild food or alcohol poisoning. Seek medical attention immediately in the case of chemical poisoning.

Location: On the ball of the foot, directly below the first toe.

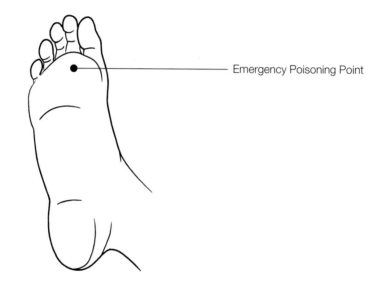

Emergency Poisoning Point

Technique: Place your fingers over the top of the person's feet for support and apply firm acupressure to the point on the sole using the thumbs. The point may be tender but maintain pressure using small rotations for several minutes. The person may feel nauseous and vomit.

HANGOVER

Encourage the person to drink plenty of fluids, especially water. Vitamin C and the B vitamins can help to restore liver function. The homoeopathic remedy Nux Vomica may also bring quick relief. Gentle exercise is beneficial and the following acupoints will help:

Large Intestine 4

Location: See page 301.

Technique: See page 301.

Benefits: Clears the head, relieves headache and helps to expel toxins from the body.

Liver 3

Location: On the top of the foot in the web between the first and second toes, just before the join of the small bones of the foot.

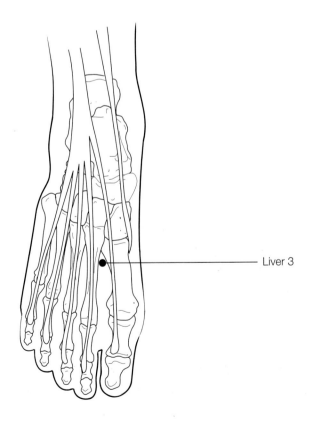

Liver 3

Technique: Place your hands under the person's feet for support and press into the point perpendicularly with your thumbs. Take care to apply pressure in the hollow between the bone and the tendons rather than on the tendons or blood vessels themselves.

Benefits: Stimulates the liver, relieves headache and aching eyes, and promotes recovery from hangover.

Note: If pregnant, see pp. 10–11.

INSECT STINGS AND BITES

If the sting has been left in the skin, remove it using tweezers or the fingernails. Do not try to squeeze the poison out of the skin, as this will only drive it deeper into the tissues. Apply a cold compress to reduce swelling and take the homoeopathic remedy Apis as soon as possible and over several hours afterwards as indicated. Homoeopathic Pyrethrum applied to the skin before going out acts as an insect repellent and can prevent insect bites. Use the following acupoints:

Urinary Bladder 65

Location: On the outside edge of the foot in the depression under the bone just beyond the join of the little toe to the foot.

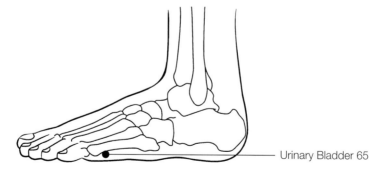

Urinary Bladder 65

Technique: Support the person's foot in your hands and locate the point using your thumbs. Apply acupressure with the nail edge of your thumbs underneath the bone and angled towards the toe.

Benefits: Reduces pain and shock from stings and helps to expel poison from the body.

If the person is shocked, add acupoints *Governor Vessel 26* and *Kidney 1*, and see Shock (below). If the person has been stung in the mouth or throat, have them rinse their mouth with cold water or suck an ice cube and remove to hospital immediately. If breathing becomes difficult, treat as for asphyxia (pp. 291–3).

See also Bites (pp. 294–5).

NOSEBLEEDS

See Nosebleeds (pp. 97–8).

SHOCK

For shock, reassure and comfort the person and keep them warm. In severe cases, lie the person down with the head low and turned to one side and the feet slightly raised to increase the blood supply to the brain. The Bach Flower Rescue Remedy can also be given for all cases of shock. Place a few drops in a glass of water for the person to sip throughout the day. Apply the following acupoints:

Governor Vessel 26

Location: In the groove below the nose, slightly more than halfway up.

Technique: Locate the point with the nail edge or fingertip of your index or middle finger or thumb. Apply acupressure lightly, pressing perpendicularly against the gums underneath.

Caution: Do not overstimulate this point if you have high blood pressure; stop immediately if you feel unwell or uncomfortable.

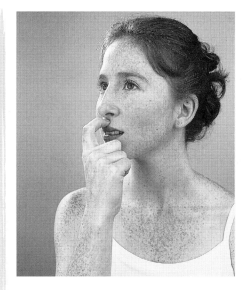

Benefits: Relieves shock and restores mental alertness.

Kidney 1

Location: A third of the way down the sole of the foot, in the depression just below the ball of the foot.

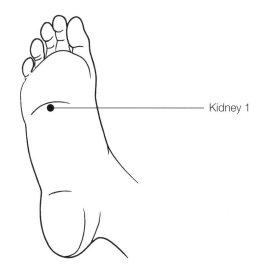

Kidney 1

Technique: Turn the sole of the person's foot upwards or sideways and support it with your fingers. Apply pressure perpendicularly, using your thumbs.

Benefits: Regulates the blood pressure, relieves shock and restores vitality to the body.

SPRAINS

Rest and raise the injured part of the body and apply an ice pack for a short time (frozen peas wrapped in a towel will do) to reduce swelling and pain. Homoeopathic Arnica will also help reduce swelling and bruising. For sprains of the ankle, use:

Urinary Bladder 60

Location: In the depression behind the ankle bone on the outside edge of the ankle.

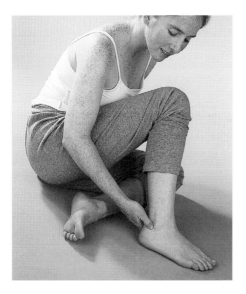

Technique: Hold the person's feet in your hands and apply pressure to the point using the index or middle finger or thumbs.

Benefits: Reduces swelling and pain of the ankle.

Note: If pregnant, see pp. 10–11.

For swelling and pain of the wrist, use:

Large Intestine 5

Location: On the thumb side of the wrist in the hollow created between the tendons when the thumb is raised.

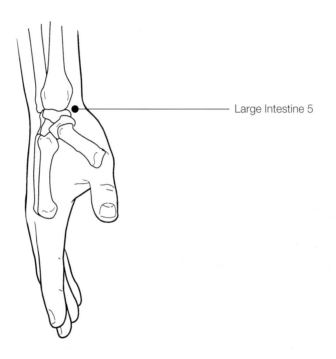

Large Intestine 5

Technique: Support the person's wrist in your hand apply pressure with your thumbs angled in the direction of the elbow.

Benefits: Reduces pain and swelling in the wrist.

See also Bruising (pp. 296–7).

Move the person to a cool place and cool the skin by sponging it gently with cold water. Apply calamine or aloe lotion and use the following acupoint. Give the person sips of water.

Urinary Bladder 65

Location: On the outside edge of the foot in the depression under the bone just beyond the join of the little toe to the foot.

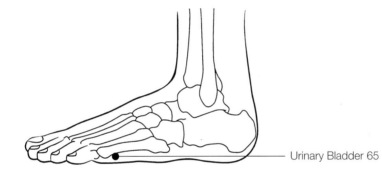

Urinary Bladder 65

Technique: Hold the person's feet in your hands and locate the point using your thumbs. Apply acupressure with the nail edge up underneath the bone and angled towards the toe.

Benefits: Helps to cool the body and reduces pain from burns.

SUNSTROKE

Lead the person to a cool place and give them sips of cold water to drink. If the person has severe cramps, due to loss of fluids and salt deficiency in the body, add half a teaspoon of salt to each pint of water. *Never* give salt water to babies or young children as their kidneys are not fully developed and this can be fatal. Use the following acupoint:

Lung 11

Location: On the outside edge of the thumb, by the corner of the thumbnail.

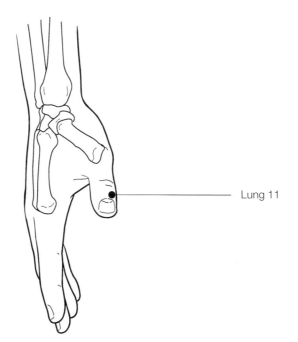

Lung 11

Technique: Support the person's thumb in your hand and apply acupressure using the nail of the opposite thumb.

Benefits: Reduces temperature and dizziness. Enhances breathing and restores mental clarity.

If the person's temperature does not return to normal, seek medical attention urgently.

See Toothache and Dental Problems (pp. 102–5).

TRAVEL SICKNESS

Before setting off on the journey, drink an infusion of ginger grated in warm water or apply finely chopped ginger to your food. Apply acupressure to the following point and continue applying it during the journey. Alternatively, wrist bands can now be bought which apply continuous pressure to this point. If travelling by car, sit in the front and focus on the road; don't try to read. If travelling by plane, adjust overhead vents so that some fresh air blows on your face. Don't travel on an empty stomach but eat light foods and drink plenty of water.

Pericardium 6

Location: Between the tendons on the inside of the arm, 3 finger widths above the wrist crease closest to the palm.

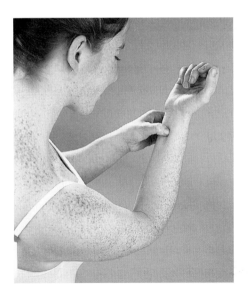

Technique: Measure up from the wrist crease to locate the point. Support the person's wrist in your hand and apply acupressure to the point using your thumb, angled downwards towards the middle finger.

Benefits: Relieves nausea and travel sickness.

See also Nausea and Travel Sickness (pp. 173–4).

List of Acupoints

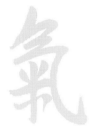

Further Reading

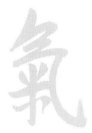

Acupressure

Jarmey, Chris, and Tindall, John, *Acupressure for Common Ailments* (Gaia Books, London, UK, 1991).

Kenyon, Dr Julian, *Acupressure Techniques: A Self-Help Guide* (Thorsons, London, UK, 1987).

Reed Gach, Michael, *Acupressure* (Piatkus, London, UK, 1992).

Reed Gach, Michael, *Arthritis Relief at Your Fingertips* (Piatkus, London, UK, 1997).

Acupuncture and the Meridians

Firebrace, Peter, and Hill, Sandra, *A Guide to Acupuncture* (Constable, London, UK, 1994).

Kaptchuk, T. J., *The Web that has no Weaver* (Contemporary, Illinois, USA, 2000).

Kenyon, Dr J. N., *Modern Techniques of Acupuncture Vols I, II and III* (Thorsons, London, UK, 1983, 1983 and 1985).

Manaka, Dr Y., and Urquhart, Dr I. A., *The Layman's Guide to Acupuncture* (Weatherhill, NY, USA, 1972).

Young, Jacqueline, *Eastern Healing: The Practical Guide to the Healing Traditions of China, India, Tibet and Japan* (Duncan Baird Publishers, London, UK, 2001).

Chelation Therapy

Collings, J., *Beat Heart Disease Without Surgery* (Thorsons, London, UK, 1995).

Eye Exercises

Bates, W. H., *Better Eyesight without Glasses* (Grafton Books, London, UK, 1987).
Benjamin, Harry, *Better Sight without Glasses* (Thorsons, London, UK, 1985).
Mansfield, P., *The Bates Method* (Vermillion, London, UK, 1995).

Food Intolerance

Brostoff, Jonathan, and Gamlin, Linda, *Food Allergies and Food Intolerance: The Complete Guide to their Identification and Treatment* (Healing Art Press, UK, 2000).
Grant, Doris, Joice, Jean, and Mills, Sir John, *Food Combining for Health* (HarperCollins, London, UK, 1993).
Marsden, Kathryn, *The Complete Book of Food Combining* (Piatkus, London, UK, 2000).

Massage and Shiatsu

Dawes, Nigel, and Harrold, Fiona, *Massage Cures: The Family Guide to Curing Common Ailments with Simple Massage Techniques* (Thorsons, London, UK, 1990).
Jarmey, Chris, *Shiatsu the Complete Guide* (HarperCollins, London, UK, 1992).
Liechti, Elaine, *The Complete Illustrated Guide to Shiatsu* (Element, London, UK, 1998).
Masunaga, Shizuto, with Ohashi, Wataru, *Zen Shiatsu: How to Harmonise Yin and Yang for Better Health* (Japan Publications, Tokyo, Japan, 1971).
Ohashi, Wataru, *Do-It-Yourself Shiatsu* (Penguin, London, UK, 2001).
Young, Jacqueline, *Self-Massage* (Thorsons, London, UK, 1992).

Mental Affirmation and Positive Thinking

Gawain, Shakti, *Creative Visualisation* (New World Library, USA, 1995), *Living in the Light* (Bantam Books, USA, 1993).
Hay, Louise, *You can Heal your Life* (Eden Grove Editions, London, UK, 1988).
Shine, Betty, *Mind Magic* (Corgi, London, UK, 1992), *Mind Waves* (Corgi, London, UK, 1994).

Natural Pregnancy

Balaskas, J., and Gordon, Y., *The Encyclopaedia of Pregnancy and Birth* (Little, Brown & Co, UK, 1992).

Balaskas, J., and Gordon Y., *New Natural Pregnancy* (Gaia Books, London, UK, 1998).

Castro, Miranda, *Homeopathy for Mother and Baby* (Macmillan, London, UK, 1992).

West, Zita, *Natural Pregnancy* (Dorling Kindersley, London, UK, 2001).

Nutritional Medicine

Chaitow, Leon, *Candida Albicans* (HarperCollins, London, UK, 1996).

Chaitow, Leon, *Natural Alternatives to Antibiotics* (HarperCollins, London, UK, 2001).

Davies, Dr Stephen, and Stewart, Dr Alan, *Nutritional Medicine: The Drug Free Guide to Better Family Health* (Pan Books, London, UK, 1987).

Hartvig, Kirsten, and Rowley, Nic, *Ten Days to Better Health* (Piatkus, London, UK, 1998).

Lazarides, Linda, *Nutritional Health Bible* (HarperCollins, London, UK, 1997).

Rowley, Nic, and Hartvig, Kirsten, *The Detox Box* (Duncan Baird, London, UK, 2000).

Qi Gong and Meridian Exercises

Chuen, Master Lam Kam, *The Way of Energy* (Gaia Books, London, UK, 1981).

Masunaga, Shizuto, and Brown, Stephen, *Zen Imagery Exercises: Meridian Exercises for Wholesome Living* (Japan Publications, Tokyo, Japan, 1987).

Young, Jacqueline, *Vital Energy: Oriental Exercises for Health and Well Being* (Hodder and Stoughton, Sevenoaks, UK, 1990).

Yoga and Meditation

Fontana, D., *The Elements of Meditation* (Element, London, UK, 1994).

Fraser, Tara, *Yoga for You* (Duncan Baird, London, UK, 2001).

H. R. and Monroe, R., *Yoga for Common Ailments* (Gaia Books, London, UK, 1990).

Sivananda Yoga Centre, *The Book of Yoga* (Ebury Press, London, UK, 1983).

Sivananda Yoga Vedanta Centre, *Yoga Mind and Body* (Dorling Kindersley, London, UK, 1996).

Useful Addresses

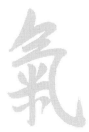

The addresses in the US, Australia and Canada were kindly provided by HarperSanFrancisco and HarperCollins Australia in order to provide a starting-point for readers in these countries. The author would like to state that she has no direct knowledge of these organizations.

Complementary Medicine Organisations

AUSTRALIA

The Australasian College of Natural Therapies
57 Foueux Street
Surry Hills, NSW 2010
Tel: 02 9218 8850
www.acnt.edu.au

The Australian Natural Therapeutic Association
31 Victoria Street
Fitzroy, Melbourne

Australian Natural Therapists Association Ltd
38 Sturt Avenue
Narrabundah
ACT, 2604
Tel: 1800 817 577
www.anta.com.au

2/5–7 Ethell Street
Kirrawee
NSW, 2022
Tel: 02 542 1466

727 Nicklin Way
QLD, 4551
Brisbane
Tel: 07 493 5113

354 Burwood Highway
Bennetswood
VIC, 3125
Tel: 03 808 9555

UNITED KINGDOM

Research Council for Complementary
Medicine (RCCM)
Suite 5, 1 Harley Street
London W1G 9QD
Tel: 0207 833 8897
www.rccm.org.uk

Foundation for Integrated Medicine
International House
59 Compton Road
London N1 2YT
Tel: 0207 688 1881
www.fimed.org

Institute for Complementary Medicine
PO Box 194
London SE16 1QZ

Council for Complementary &
Alternative Medicine
Suite D, Park House
206–208 Latimer Road
London W10 6RE

UNITED STATES OF AMERICA

Association of Health Practitioners
PO Box 5007
Durango, CO 81301
Tel: 303 259 1091

Acupressure/Shiatsu Practitioners

UNITED KINGDOM

British School of Shiatsu-do
97–99 Seven Sisters Road
London N7 7QP
Tel: 0207 483 3776
www.shiatsu-do.co.uk

Shen Tao Foundation
Middle Piccadilly Natural Healing Centre
Holwell, Sherbourne
Dorset
Tel: 01963 23302

The Shiatsu Society, UK
Eastlands Court
St. Peter's Road
Rugby
Warwickshire
CV21 3QP
Tel: 01788 555051
www.shiatsu.org

UNITED STATES OF AMERICA

Acupressure Institute
1533 Shattuck Avenue
Berkeley, CA 94709
Tel: 510 845 1059
www.acupressure.com

Southeast Institute of Oriental Medicine
10506 N. Kendall Drive
Miami, FL 33176
Tel: 305 595 9500
www.seiom.com

Acupuncturists

(Many also practise acupressure.)

CANADA

Acupuncture Foundation of Canada
Institute (AFCI)
2131 Lawrence Avenue East
Suite 204
Scarborough
Ontario M1R 5RG
Tel: 416 752 3988
www.afcinstitute.com

UNITED KINGDOM
British Acupuncture Council
63 Jeddo Road
London W12 9HQ
Tel: 0208 735 0400
www.acupuncture.org.uk

UNITED STATES OF AMERICA
Acupuncture International Association
2330 S. Brentwood Boulevard
St Louis, MO 63144
Tel: 314 961 2300

American Association of Acupuncture
& Oriental Medicine
4101 Lake Boone Trail
Suite 201
Raleigh, NC 27607
Tel: 919 787 5181

Allergy and Environmental Medicine Specialists

AUSTRALIA

The Allergy Association of Australia
PO Box 214
North Beach, WA 6020
Tel: 08 9246 1595

The Allergy Association of South Australia
PO Box 104
North Adelaide, SA 5006
Tel: 08 8214 1548

UNITED KINGDOM

British Society of Allergy
& Environmental Medicine
Burghwood Clinic
34 Brighton Road, Banstead
Surrey SM17 1BS
Tel: 01737 361177

Centre for the Study of Complementary
Medicine
51 Bedford Place
Southampton SO1 2DG
Tel: 01703 334752
www.complemed.co.uk

UNITED STATES OF AMERICA

American Academy of Environmental
Medicine
7701 East Kellogg
Suite 625
Wichita
Kansas 67207
Tel: 316 684 5500
www.aaem.com

National centre for diagnosis
and treatment of allergies.
UCLA Medical Center
10833 Leconte Avenue
Los Angeles
CA 90024–1602
Tel: 310 825 9111
www.healthcare.ucla.edu

Bach Flower Remedies

The Dr Edward Bach Centre
Mount Vernon
Sotwell
Wallingford
Oxfordshire OX10 0PZ

Bates Eye Method

The Bates Association of Great Britain
PO Box 25
Shoreham-by-Sea
West Sussex BN43 6ZF

Herbalists

AUSTRALIA
The National Herbalists' Association
of Australia
33 Reserve Street
Annandale
NSW 2038
Tel: 02 9560 7077
www.nhaa.org.au

UNITED KINGDOM
The National Institute of Medical Herbalists
56 Longbrook Street
Exeter
Devon EX4 6AH
Tel: 01392 426022

UNITED STATES OF AMERICA
American Botanical Council
PO Box 144345
Austin, TX 78720
Tel: 512 926 4900
www.herbalgram.org

American Herbalists Guild
1931 Gaddis Road
Canton, GA 30115
Tel: 770 751 6021
www.americanherbalistsguild.com

Homoeopaths

AUSTRALIA
The Australian Federation of
Homoeopaths
10 Coles Street
4054 Arana Hills
NSW
Tel: 61 738510456

Australian Homoeopathic Association
44 Colton Avenue
Magill, SA 5072
Tel: 61 883327433

UNITED KINGDOM
British Homoeopathic Association
15 Clerkenwell Close
London EC1R 0AA
Tel: 0207 566 7800
www.trusthomeopathy.org

UNITED STATES OF AMERICA
International Foundation for Homeopathy
2366 Eastlake Avenue East
Suite 301
Seattle, WA 98102
Tel: 206 324 8230

National Center for Homeopathy
801 N. Fairfax Street
Suite 306
Alexandria, VA 22314
Tel: 703 548 7790
www.homeopathic.org

Homoeopathic Pharmacies

UNITED KINGDOM
Ainsworths Homoeopathic Pharmacy
36 New Cavendish Street
London W1M 7LH
Tel: 0207 935 5330
www.ainsworths.com

UNITED STATES OF AMERICA
Homeopathic Educational Services
2124 Kittredge Street
Berkeley, CA 90061
Tel: 800 624 9659

Natural Pregnancy

UNITED KINGDOM
Active Birth Centre
25 Bickerton Road
London N19 5JT
Tel: 0207 482 5554
www.activebirthcentre.com

Splashdown
17 Wellington Terrace
Harrow-on-the Hill
Middlesex HA1 3EP
Tel: 0208 422 9308
www.splashdown.org.uk

UNITED STATES OF AMERICA
The International Association for
Childbirth at Home
PO Box 430
Glendale, CA 91209
Tel: 213 663 4996

International Childbirth Education
Association
PO Box 20048
Minneapolis, MN 55420
Tel: 952 854 8660
www.icea.org

La Leche League International
PO Box 4079
Schaumburg, IL 60168–4079
Tel: 847 519 7730
www.lalecheleague.org

Naturopaths

UNITED KINGDOM
British Naturopathic and
Osteopathic Association
Goswell House
2 Goswell Road
Somerset BA16 0JG
Tel: 01458 840072
www.naturopathy.org.uk

UNITED STATES OF AMERICA
American Association of
Naturopathic Physicians
8201 Greensboro Drive
Suite 300
McLean, VA 22102
Tel: 703 610 9037
www.naturopathic.org

Nutritional Therapy

UNITED KINGDOM
Society for the Promotion of
Nutritional Medicine
PO Box 47
Heathfield
East Sussex TN21 82X

UNITED STATES OF AMERICA
Nutritional Health Alliance
PO Box 267
Farmingdale, NY 11735
Tel: 516 249 7070

Osteopaths

AUSTRALIA
The Australian Academy of Osteopathy
7th Floor
235 Macquarie Street
Sydney
NSW 2000
Tel: 233 1655

UNITED KINGDOM
European School of Osteopathy
104 Tonbridge Road
Maidstone
Kent ME16 8SL
Tel: 01622 671558

General Council and Register
of Osteopaths
56 London Street
Reading
Berkshire RG1 4SQ
Tel: 01734 576585

Osteopathic Information Service
PO Box 2074
Reading
Berkshire RG1 4YR

UNITED STATES OF AMERICA
American Academy of Osteopathy
2630 Airport Road
Colorado Springs, CO 80910

The American Osteopathic Association
142 E Ontario Street
Chicago, IL 60611
Tel: 312 280 5800

Yoga

UNITED KINGDOM
British Wheel of Yoga
1 Hamilton Place
Boston Road
Sleaford
Lincolnshire NG34 7ES
Tel: 01529 306851

Yoga for Health Foundation
Ickwell Bury
Nr Biggleswade
Bedfordshire SG18 9EF
Tel: 01767 627271

UNITED STATES OF AMERICA
California Yoga Teachers Association
380 Stevens Avenue
Suite 115
Solano Beach, CA 92075
Tel: 800 395 8075

Index

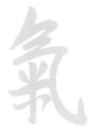

Practical Reiki
A step-by-step guide

Mari Hall

Practical Reiki is a fully illustrated guide to Reiki, the ancient form of harmonization through the laying on of hands. This method of transmitting universal energy can bring great relief to the recipient; not just in the physical body, but also on an emotional and spiritual level.

The most common effects of a Reiki session are deep relaxation and a sense of inner peace. This creates an ideal environment for the body to maximize its natural healing processes. Reiki can be used safely at any time, in any place and for anything – from problems with conceiving to alleviating the pain of terminal illness.

Includes:
- Spiritual principles of Reiki
- Self treatment
- Treating others
- Reiki and the emotions
- Using Reiki in conjunction with other healing methods

Reflexology for Women

Nicola Hall

Reflexology for Women **is a fully illustrated guide to healing the body. Reflexology is a gentle form of natural healing and involves massaging the 'reflex' areas in the feet and hands, which correspond to various parts of the body. As well as being relaxing, reflexology is an effective treatment for many health problems and disorders.**

This book deals with the basic health concerns and common problems that affect women through various stages of their lives, including:
- menstruation
- pregnancy
- menopause
- fluid retention
- breast problems
- cystitis
- skin problems
- depression

Reflexology for Women is essential reading for health-conscious women and gives a simple introduction to the art of reflexology.

Big Book of Ch'i
An exploration of energy, form and spirit

Paul Wildish

Fabulously illustrated with colour photographs throughout, *The Big Book of Ch'i* takes a fascinating look at the origins of ch'i and the wide range of practices that focus on ch'i, our living essence – from martial and healing arts to feng shui. It teaches us ways to awaken this energy and fulfil our true potential.

In the West, we give little thought to 'energy', but the understanding of our energy, or life force, is the basis of virtually all Eastern healing and exercise practices. The Chinese believe that understanding and balancing the flow of this 'ch'i' energy is essential for well-being.

Whether your interest is in healing, martial arts or feng shui, *The Big Book of Ch'i* will bring you to a profound understanding of this vital energy and how to access and channel it for your own well-being.